TRAILS OF THE
ANGELES
10TH
EDITION

100 HIKES IN THE SAN GABRIEL MOUNTAINS

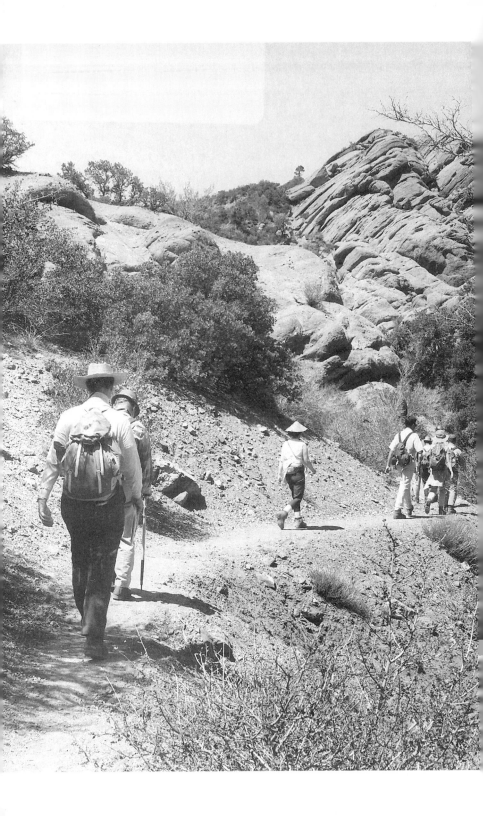

TRAILS OF THE
ANGELES

10TH EDITION

00 HIKES IN THE SAN GABRIEL MOUNTAINS

DAVID HARRIS

Prior editions by JOHN W. ROBINSON

WILDERNESS PRESS ... *on the trail since 1967*

TRAILS OF THE ANGELES: 100 HIKES IN THE SAN GABRIEL MOUNTAINS

10th Edition 2021
Copyright © 2021 by David Harris
Copyright © 2005 and 2013 by Doug Christiansen
Copyright © 1971, 1973, 1976, 1979, 1984, 1990, and 1998 by John W. Robinson

Front cover photos copyright © 2021 by David Harris (top: Mount Waterman summit rocks;
    bottom: Baldy North Backbone
Interior photos by David Harris, except where noted
Frontispiece: Trail to Devil's Punchbowl (see Hike 69)
Pocket map design: Chris Salcedo/Blue Gecko, using data from John W. Robinson, Laurence Jones,
    David Harris, Doug Christiansen, and U.S. Geological Survey topos
Cover design and back cover map: Scott McGrew
Book design: Annie Long

Manufactured in the United States of America

Library of Congress Cataloging-in-Publication Data

Names: Harris, David Money, author.
Title: Trails of the Angeles : 100 hikes in the San Gabriel Mountains / David Harris.
Description: 10th edition. | Birmingham, AL : Wilderness Press, 2021. | Revised edition
    of: Trails of the Angeles : 100 hikes in the San Gabriels / John W. Robinson with Doug
    Christiansen. Ninth edition. 2013. | Summary: "This updated guidebook details 100 hikes
    in the San Gabriel Mountains, from one-hour strolls to five-day backcountry trips" —
    Provided by publisher.
Identifiers: LCCN 2020040267 (pbk.) | LCCN 2020040268 (ebook) | ISBN 9781643590295
    (pbk.) | ISBN 9781643590301 (ebook)
Subjects: LCSH: Hiking—California—San Gabriel Mountains—Guidebooks. | Trails—
    California—San Gabriel Mountains—Guidebooks. | San Gabriel Mountains (Calif.)—
    Guidebooks.
Classification: LCC GV199.42.C22 S277 2021 (pbk.) | LCC GV199.42.C22 (ebook) |
    DDC 796.5109794/93—dc23
LC record available at lccn.loc.gov/2020040267
LC ebook record available at lccn.loc.gov/2020040268

🎯 WILDERNESS PRESS

An imprint of AdventureKEEN
2204 First Ave. S., Suite 102
Birmingham, AL 35233
800-443-7227; fax 205-326-1012

Visit wildernesspress.com for a complete listing of our books and for ordering information. Contact us
at our website, at facebook.com/wildernesspress1967, or at twitter.com/wilderness1967 with questions
or comments. To find out more about who we are and what we're doing, visit blog.wildernesspress.com.

Distributed by Publishers Group West

SAFETY NOTICE Although Wilderness Press and the author have made every attempt to ensure that
the information in this book is accurate at press time, they are not responsible for any loss, damage,
injury, or inconvenience that may occur to anyone while using this book. You are responsible for your
own safety and health while in the wilderness. The fact that a trail is described in this book does not
mean that it will be safe for you. Be aware that trail conditions can change from day to day. Always
check local conditions and know your own limitations.

▪ Contents ▪

▪ 100 HIKES IN THE SAN GABRIEL MOUNTAINS

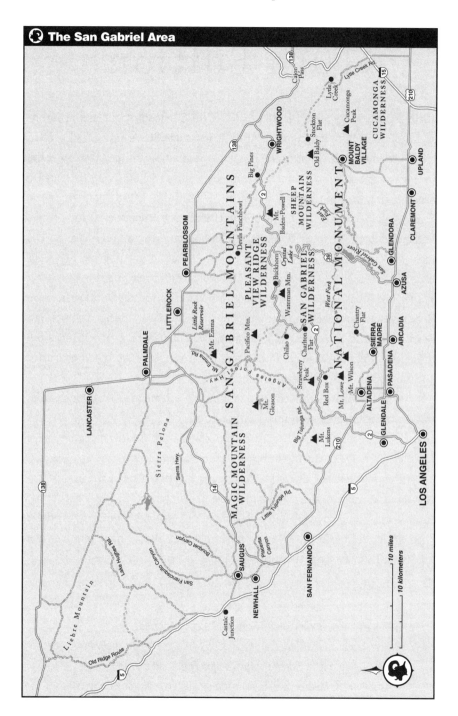

The San Gabriel Area

Preface to the 10th Edition

JOHN ROBINSON, SOUTHERN CALIFORNIA'S legendary guidebook author and mountain historian, died in April 2018 at age 88. A native Californian, he served in the army during the Korean War and then studied history at the University of Southern California before becoming a schoolteacher. Robinson began hiking with the Sierra Club in the 1950s and co-led the first trip of the Sierra Peaks Section in 1956. He founded the "Sierra Echo," the section's newsletter, and went on to write hiking guidebooks and mountain histories. His most famous hiking guidebooks are this one, *Trails of the Angeles,* first published in 1971, and *San Bernardino Mountain Trails,* first published in 1972. Wilderness Press has kept both in continuous print for nearly 50 years now. Robinson also wrote the most comprehensive histories of the San Gabriel, San Bernardino, and San Jacinto Mountains, meticulously researched tomes full of historical photos that are fascinating for anyone wondering who roamed our mountains in bygone days.

When Robinson retired from guidebook writing in 2005, Doug Christiansen revised the eighth and ninth editions of *Trails of the Angeles.* Now that Christiansen's career has taken him away from Southern California, I have the privilege of tracing Robinson's footsteps through the San Gabriels.

This revision has proved to be the most substantial in the book's history. For this edition, I have rehiked every hike in the book, mostly in the past three years. Some have burned or become impassable. I have merged others with closely related trips. A few were simply dull. Thus, I have removed the following 18 hikes from the ninth edition:

2. Sawmill Ridge to Gillette Mine: *Unmaintained and overgrown*
6. Dagger Flat: *Burned in the Sand Fire and brushy*
8. Barley Flats: *Burned in the Station Fire and vanished*
9. Tom Lucas Trail: *Burned in the Station Fire and a nasty bushwhack*
10. Messenger Flats: *Burned in the Station Fire; road closed*
13. Grizzly Flat: *Merged with nearby trip up Lukens via Stone Canyon*

18. Bear Canyon Trail Camp: *Merged with Bear Canyon Traverse*
37. Strawberry Peak Traverse: *Merged with Strawberry Peak*
42. Spruce Grove Trail Camp: *Merged with Mount Zion Loop*
46. West Fork: *Trip unclear and closely related to other West Fork trips*
49. Mount Bliss: *Uncompelling fire-road walk with poor trailhead parking*
52. Devore and West Fork: *Merged with West Fork Trail Camp*
54. Big Tujunga Narrows: *Canyoneering trip rather than a hike*
55. Mount Gleason: *Road closed since Station Fire*
62. Little Rock Creek: *Unclear; merged with nearby trips*
72. West Fork San Gabriel River: *Paved road walk ending at a fence*
78. Baden-Powell from Crystal Lake: *Replaced with a better loop*
87. Upper Fish Fork: *Unmaintained and overgrown*

In their place, I am happy to have added a delightful set of new hikes, including a mix of waterfalls, newly reopened trails, family-friendly rambles, and epic adventures.

5. Whitney Canyon: *Waterfall*
7. Trail Canyon Falls: *Waterfall and the best part of the Tom Lucas hike*
21. Eaton Canyon Falls: *The most popular waterfall in the San Gabriels*
41. Monrovia Canyon Falls: *Waterfall*
46. Vetter Mountain: *Family-friendly hike to historic fire-lookout site*
53. Winston Peak: *An easy summit in the Angeles High Country*
58. Kratka Ridge: *Splendid views on a short stretch of the Pacific Crest Trail*
64. High Desert Loop: *A backpacking trip or long day hike that has it all*
70. Mount Islip South Ridge: *A scenic trail on Islip reopened by volunteers*
74. Silver Moccasin Trail: *The best 50 miles through the Angeles*
79. Rattlesnake Peak: *A fun route on a wild and rugged mountain*
81. San Antonio Ridge: *The hardest traverse in the Angeles*
84. Jackson Lake Loop: *An enjoyable ramble in the woods*
85. Big Dalton Mystic Loop: *A short but vigorous workout in the canyon*
87. Claremont Hills Wilderness Park: *The most heavily visited wilderness park*
88. Etiwanda Falls: *Waterfall in a recently opened nature preserve*
89. Stoddard Peak: *Moderate peak climb with great views*
91. San Antonio Falls: *Waterfall*

I have also added variations to many of the existing and new hikes to help customize the trips to your hiking preferences.

I have endeavored to keep Robinson's poetic prose wherever possible. Most of the hikes have been edited substantially as trails have changed and more information has become available. I have updated driving directions to be easier to follow and have simplified the names of most hikes. The United States Geological Survey (USGS) maps recommended in previous editions are becoming outdated and inconvenient to use, so I have replaced them with commercial maps that are more accurate, more easily available, and less expensive. I also provide GPS data for all the hikes online at etrails.net and through a free iOS app called eTrails.

In 2014, President Barack Obama designated the 346,177-acre San Gabriel Mountains National Monument, encompassing much of the high country in the Angeles National Forest and managed by the U.S. Forest Service. At the time of this writing, the monument designation has not brought significant new resources or major changes to the trail network, but over time it may facilitate improvements.

Acknowledgments

I WOULD LIKE TO THANK Werner Zorman and Elizabeth Thomas for company in Thursday Morning Hiking Club. My sons joined me for many days of field work. Andrew Mitchell, Richard Wilmer, and Zachary Behrens clarified permit information. Tom Chester, Kristen Sabo, Kyle Kuns, Melissa Tovar, and David Baumgartner shared their knowledge of the trails.

Kate Johnson was the project editor, and Annie Long did the book layout. The remaining errors are my own.

Summary of Hikes

NUMBER	HIKE	DIFFICULTY**	DISTANCE (miles)	ELEVATION GAIN (feet)	TRAIL TYPE	PERMITS	DOGS ALLOWED	GOOD FOR KIDS	MOUNTAIN BIKING	BACKPACKING
1	Liebre Mountain	M	7	1,700	Out & back	N/A	✓			✓
2	Fish Canyon Narrows	M	10	800	Out & back	N/A	✓		✓	✓
3	Sierra Pelona	M	6	1,300	Out & back	N/A	✓			
4	Placerita Canyon Park	M	7	1,800	Loop	N/A	✓			
5	Whitney Canyon	E	3.4	300	Out & back	N/A	✓	✓	✓	
6	Yerba Buena Ridge	M	4.6	1,400	Out & back	N/A	✓		✓	
7	Trail Canyon Falls	M	4.5	1,000	Out & back	N/A	✓	✓		✓
8	Mount Lukens via Stone Canyon Trail	S	8	3,300	Out & back	AP	✓			
9	Condor Peak	S	15	3,400	Out & back	N/A	✓			
10	Mount Lukens via Haines Canyon Trail	S	10	2,800	Out & back	N/A	✓		✓	
11	Lower Arroyo Seco	E	5	300	Out & back	N/A	✓	✓	✓	✓
12	Down the Arroyo Seco	M	10	-2,700	Out & back	AP	✓		✓	✓
13	Switzer Falls	E	3.6	700	Out & back	AP	✓	✓	✓	
14	Dawn Mine	M	6	1,500	Loop	N/A	✓	✓		
15	Millard Canyon Falls	E	1.2	250	Out & back	AP	✓	✓		
16	Brown Mountain Loop	S	12	3,000	Loop	N/A	✓			
17	Mount Lowe Trail Camp from Sunset Ridge	S	11	2,600	Loop	N/A	✓		✓	✓
18	Mount Lowe Railway Loop Tour	S	11	2,800	Loop	N/A	✓			✓
19	Echo Mountain	M	5	1,400	Out & back	N/A	✓			
20	Rubio Canyon	E	1.5	200	Out & back	N/A	✓	✓		
21	Eaton Canyon Falls	E	3.5	500	Out & back	N/A	✓	✓		
22	Henninger Flats	M	5.5	1,400	Out & back	N/A	✓	✓	✓	✓
23	Mount Wilson Toll Road*	M	9	-4,500	Out & back	N/A	✓		✓	✓

*Hike was affected by the Bobcat Fire. See page 15 for more information.

**E = Easy; M = Moderate; S = Strenuous

SUMMARY OF HIKES

NUMBER	HIKE	DIFFICULTY**	DISTANCE (miles)	ELEVATION GAIN (feet)	TRAIL TYPE	PERMITS	DOGS ALLOWED	GOOD FOR KIDS	MOUNTAIN BIKING	BACKPACKING
24	Idlehour Trail	S	14	4,100	↗	N/A	🐕			🥾
25	San Gabriel Peak from Red Box	M	4	1,400	↗	N/A	🐕			
26	Mount Lowe from Eaton Saddle	E	3	500	↗	N/A	🐕	🧍		
27	Mount Lowe Trail Camp from Eaton Saddle	M	6	1,500	↺	N/A	🐕		⦿	🥾
28	San Gabriel Peak from Eaton Saddle	M	3	1,000	↗	N/A	🐕	🧍		
29	Bear Canyon Traverse	M	8	-2,700	↗	AP	🐕			🥾
30	Jones Peak	M	6	2,300	↗	N/A	🐕			
31	Josephine Peak	M	8	1,900	↗	N/A	🐕		⦿	
32	Strawberry Peak	M	7	2,600	↗	N/A				
33	Strawberry Meadow	M	9	1,600	↗	AP	🐕		⦿	🥾
34	Orchard Camp*	M	7	2,000	↗	N/A	🐕			🥾
35	Mount Wilson via Old Mount Wilson Trail*	M	7	-4,500	↗	AP	🐕			🥾
36	Sturtevant Falls*	E	3.3	600	↗	AP	🐕	🧍		
37	Mount Zion Loop*	M	8.5	2,000	↺	AP	🐕			🥾
38	Mount Wilson via Winter Creek*	S	6	3,600	↗	AP	🐕			
39	Mount Wilson via Sturtevant Camp*	S	7	3,900	↗	AP	🐕			🥾
40	Gabrielino National Recreation Trail*	S	28	4,800	↗	AP	🐕			🥾
41	Monrovia Canyon Falls*	E	2.6	600	↗	$	🐕	🧍		
42	Ben Overturff Trail*	M	7	1,700	↺	N/A	🐕		⦿	
43	Fish Canyon Falls	E	3.4	600	↗	N/A	🐕	🧍		

*Hike was affected by the Bobcat Fire. See page 15 for more information.
**E = Easy; M = Moderate; S = Strenuous

SUMMARY OF HIKES

NUMBER	HIKE	DIFFICULTY**	DISTANCE (miles)	ELEVATION GAIN (feet)	TRAIL TYPE	PERMITS	DOGS ALLOWED	GOOD FOR KIDS	MOUNTAIN BIKING	BACKPACKING
44	Kenyon DeVore Trail to West Fork Trail Camp*	M	8	2,800	↗	N/A	🐕			🎒
45	Shortcut Canyon to West Fork Trail Camp*	M	7	1,800	↗	N/A	🐕			🎒
46	Vetter Mountain*	E	3.6	700	○	N/A	🐕	👥		
47	Pacifico Mountain	M	10	1,700	↗	N/A	🐕			🎒
48	Devils Canyon*	M	6	1,500	↗	AP	🐕			🎒
49	Mount Hillyer	M	6	1,000	○	N/A	🐕	👥		🎒
50	Twin Peaks and Mount Waterman Traverse*	S	13	4,000	↗	AP	🐕			
51	Mount Waterman from Buckhorn*	M	6	1,300	↗	N/A	🐕			
52	Cloudburst to Cooper Canyon Falls to Buckhorn*	M	4.5	800	↗	AP	🐕	👥		🎒
53	Winston Peak*	E	1.2	500	↗	N/A	🐕	👥		
54	Pleasant View Ridge*	S	12	3,500	↗	AP	🐕			🎒
55	Eagles Roost Picnic Area to Cooper Canyon Falls*	M	7	1,100	↗	AP	🐕			
56	Mount Williamson*	M	3.6	1,400	↗	N/A	🐕			🎒
57	Williamson–Burkhart Traverse*	S	12	3,500	○	N/A	🐕			🎒
58	Kratka Ridge*	E	1.8	400	↗	AP	🐕	👥		
59	Burkhart Trail*	S	14	3,200	↗	N/A	🐕			
60	Devil's Punchbowl Natural Area and Nature Center*	E	1.2	300	○	N/A	🐕	👥		
61	Devils Chair*	M	5.5	1,300	↗	N/A	🐕	👥		🎒
62	South Fork Trail*	M	10	2,100	↗	N/A	🐕			
63	Manzanita Trail	M	11	2,400	↗	N/A	🐕			

*Hike was affected by the Bobcat Fire. See page 15 for more information.
**E = Easy; M = Moderate; S = Strenuous

SUMMARY OF HIKES

NUMBER	HIKE	DIFFICULTY**	DISTANCE (miles)	ELEVATION GAIN (feet)	TRAIL TYPE	PERMITS	DOGS ALLOWED	GOOD FOR KIDS	MOUNTAIN BIKING	BACKPACKING
64	High Desert Loop*	S	23	5,500	loop	N/A	✓			✓
65	Smith Mountain	M	7	1,800	out-and-back	N/A	✓			
66	Bear Creek*	S	11	1,100	out-and-back	AP	✓			✓
67	Lewis Falls	E	1	300	out-and-back	N/A	✓	✓		
68	Mount Islip via Windy Gap*	M	7	2,500	loop	N/A	✓			✓
69	Mount Islip from Islip Saddle*	M	7	1,500	out-and-back	AP	✓			✓
70	Mount Islip South Ridge*	S	10	2,800	loop	N/A	✓			✓
71	Mount Hawkins Loop	S	13	3,700	loop	N/A	✓			✓
72	Throop Peak*	M	4	1,200	out-and-back	N/A	✓			✓
73	Mount Baden-Powell from Vincent Gap	M	8	2,800	out-and-back	AP	✓			✓
74	Silver Moccasin Trail*	S	52	14,600	out-and-back	AP	✓			✓
75	Big Horn Mine	E	4	500	out-and-back	AP	✓		✓	
76	Upper East Fork	M	8	2,000	out-and-back	AP	✓			✓
77	Bridge to Nowhere	M	10	800	out-and-back	AP, WP	✓			✓
78	Up the East Fork	S	16	4,500	out-and-back	AP, WP	✓			✓
79	Rattlesnake Peak	S	9.5	4,000	loop	N/A	✓			
80	Iron Mountain	S	14	6,200	out-and-back	AP, WP	✓			
81	San Antonio Ridge	S	16	6,000	out-and-back	AP, WP	✓			
82	Mount Baldy North Backbone Traverse	S	11	5,100	out-and-back	N/A	✓			✓
83	Blue Ridge Trail	E	5	1,300	out-and-back	N/A	✓	✓	✓	✓
84	Jackson Lake Loop	M	7	1,300	loop	AP	✓			
85	Big Dalton Mystic Loop	M	3	1,300	loop	N/A	✓			

*Hike was affected by the Bobcat Fire. See page 15 for more information.

**E = Easy; M = Moderate; S = Strenuous

SUMMARY OF HIKES

NUMBER	HIKE	DIFFICULTY**	DISTANCE (miles)	ELEVATION GAIN (feet)	TRAIL TYPE	PERMITS	DOGS ALLOWED	GOOD FOR KIDS	MOUNTAIN BIKING	BACKPACKING
86	Marshall Canyon Loop	M	4.5	800	Loop	N/A	🐕	👪		
87	Claremont Hills Wilderness Park	M	5	900	Loop	$	🐕	👪		
88	Etiwanda Falls	M	5	1,200	Loop	N/A		👪		
89	Stoddard Peak	M	6	1,000	Out-and-back	N/A	🐕			
90	Sunset Peak	M	6	1,200	Out-and-back	N/A	🐕		⊕	🎒
91	San Antonio Falls	E	1.2	200	Out-and-back	N/A	🐕	👪		
92	Mount Baldy via Devils Backbone	M	6	2,300	Out-and-back	$				🎒
93	Mount Baldy via Bear Ridge	S	10	5,800	Out-and-back	N/A	🐕			🎒
94	Mount Baldy Loop	S	10	3,900	Loop	N/A	🐕			🎒
95	Stockton Flat to Baldy Notch	M	8	1,700	Out-and-back	N/A	🐕		⊕	
96	The Three Ts	M	10	2,000	One-way	AP	🐕			🎒
97	Icehouse Saddle from Icehouse Canyon	M	7	2,600	Out-and-back	AP	🐕			🎒
98	Ontario Peak	S	12	3,800	Out-and-back	AP	🐕			🎒
99	Cucamonga Peak	S	12	4,000	Out-and-back	AP, WP	🐕			🎒
100	Icehouse Saddle from Lytle Creek	S	12	3,600	Out-and-back	AP, WP	🐕			🎒

**E = Easy; M = Moderate; S = Strenuous

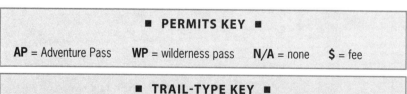

■ **PERMITS KEY** ■

AP = Adventure Pass   **WP** = wilderness pass   **N/A** = none   **$** = fee

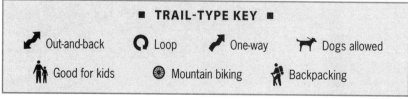

■ **TRAIL-TYPE KEY** ■

Out-and-back   Loop   One-way   Dogs allowed
Good for kids   Mountain biking   Backpacking

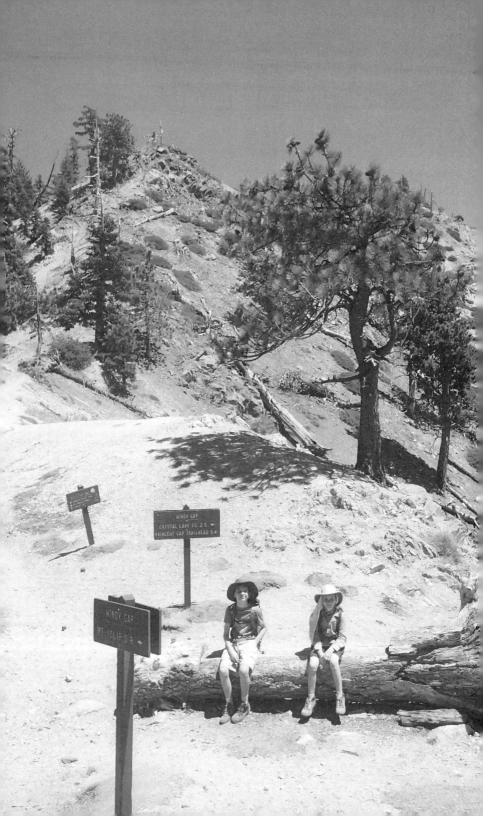

• Introduction •

"THERE IS NO EXERCISE so beneficial, physically, mentally, or morally, nothing which gives so much of living for so little cost, as hiking our mountain and hill trails and sleeping under the stars."

So wrote the late Will Thrall—explorer, historian, author, and protector of the San Gabriel Mountains of Southern California. Thrall's philosophy certainly applies today, in this age of high-pressure, rapid-paced urban life that engulfs so many Southern Californians. Fortunately, there are mountains practically in the backyard of Los Angeles that offer the harried city dweller a refreshing change of pace. Here, amid forest, chaparral, and stream, you can redeem and revitalize yourself in nature's unhurried environment. Traveling a wooded trail or scrambling along a rocky hillside, you can find solitude and gain perspective; you will come to discover the true value of wilderness to a civilization that too often places artificial values before real ones.

More than 135 years ago, in 1877, naturalist John Muir sampled the San Gabriels, found them wild and trailless, and described the range as "more rigidly inaccessible . . . than any other I ever attempted to penetrate." Great change has come to the San Gabriels since Muir's excursion. This once-primitive high country that he so vividly described in his classic *The Mountains of California* is today crisscrossed with paved highways, unpaved side roads, trails, and firebreaks. Yet wilderness is here for anyone who will leave behind pavement and campground to seek it on the numerous footpaths within range.

This guidebook represents a concerted effort to acquaint Southern Californians with the intimate parts of the San Gabriels—the regions away from highways and byways where nature remains relatively undisturbed. One hundred hiking trips take the reader and prospective hiker into almost every nook and cranny of the range. They vary from easy one-hour strolls to all-day and overnight rambles involving many miles of walking and many elevation changes, from excursions to satisfy novice hikers to challenging ones for veteran adventurers. For history buffs, there are tours of the Mount Lowe Railway and the Echo Mountain ruins; for nature

OPPOSITE: *Windy Gap (see Hike 68)*

1

lovers, there are samplings of five wilderness areas, forever left to their natural states; for peak baggers, there are routes up almost all of the major summits of the range.

The San Gabriels are laced with trails and fire roads—some well maintained and easy to follow, others nearly forgotten due to erosion and overgrowth. The great majority of trips in this guidebook are on maintained trails and should offer no problems to the hiker. However, there are a handful of cross-country excursions and trailless peak climbs in regions well worth visiting but not served by standard routes. For these trips, directions have been presented in greater detail.

The author has rewalked, recorded, and researched all the trips in this volume, most of them in recent years. Every effort has been made to present the information as accurately and as explicitly as possible. Nevertheless, the prospective hiker should be aware that several factors—some of them unique to the Southern California mountains—may make some of this information out of date in an amazingly short time. The first is the rapid growth of chaparral—the rigid, thorny brush that covers 80% of San Gabriel mountain slopes. A trail through this brushy maze, if not continually maintained, can become overgrown and virtually impassable in three years or fewer. Second is fire, the danger of which is extreme during late summer and fall when the chaparral becomes tinder-dry. Fire denudes hillsides of vegetation, leaving them subject to dirt slippage and rockslides. Third is flood. Winter rainfall is generally moderate in the Southern California mountains (compared to the Sierra Nevada and other northern ranges), but every few years, deluges occur that are particularly destructive to canyon trails. On fire-ravaged hillsides, water erosion can be severe, obliterating large sections of trail. Last is the continual reworking, regrading, and rebuilding of maintained trails by the U.S. Forest Service and volunteer conservation groups. Sometimes part of a trail is redirected along a different route or road closures require different origination points. Such changes will probably affect only a few of the trips described herein, but if you are unfamiliar with the area in which you plan to hike, it is best to inquire at a ranger station before the trip.

To inquire about fire conditions, and for general questions concerning forest entry, contact the following U.S. Forest Service facilities:

Monday–Friday:

ANGELES NATIONAL FOREST HEADQUARTERS 626-574-1613
LOS ANGELES GATEWAY RANGER DISTRICT 818-899-1900
SAN GABRIEL MOUNTAINS NATIONAL MONUMENT 626-335-1251

Saturday–Sunday:

MOUNT BALDY VISITOR CENTER 909-982-2829
GRASSY HOLLOW VISITOR CENTER 626-821-6737

This book is titled *Trails of the Angeles* because 95% of the San Gabriel Mountains are within Angeles National Forest. However, the eastern end of the range—from the great Baldy–Telegraph–Ontario Ridge to Cajon Pass—is in San Bernardino National Forest. This section boasts some of the finest high country in the mountains, and it has been included because it belongs here better than with the topographically different San Bernardino Mountains several miles east. (Refer to Wilderness Press's *San Bernardino Mountain Trails* for 100 trips in the latter range.) This book also includes several popular hikes in the canyons at the base of the San Gabriels; these are mostly administered by city or county governments rather than by the Angeles National Forest.

The trips listed here are just a beginning. Far more than 100 hikes are possible in the San Gabriels, crisscrossed as these mountains are by walking routes. Furthermore, various combinations of the routes described here are possible, particularly if you can arrange for car shuttles. You could spend a decade rambling through the range and still not have completely explored the mountains.

We hope that this guidebook will give you the knowledge that can make an outing in the San Gabriels an enjoyable and meaningful experience. Learn and heed forest regulations, follow route directions, become familiar with the area, have proper equipment, and use good sense. Never leave the trailhead without this preparation. The mountains are no place to travel alone, unbriefed, ill-equipped, or in poor condition. Enter their portals with the enthusiasm of adventure tempered with respect, forethought, and common sense. The mountains belong to those who are wise as well as willing.

The San Gabriel Mountains

AS LONG AS HUMANS have lived in the Los Angeles Basin, we have looked at the San Gabriel Mountains. Whether phantomlike behind a veil of brownish haze, sharply etched against a blue winter sky, or playing hide-and-seek with billowing clouds, they are a familiar scene on the northern skyline.

San Gabriel ridgelines are sinuous rather than jagged, the summits rounded rather than angular, and the slopes tapered rather than sheer. Although they present a formidable barrier to north–south travel, their elevations and topographical features do not compare with the sky-piercing crags of the Sierra Nevada.

The San Gabriels form a great roof over the Southern California coastal lowlands, covering an area that reaches from seaward slopes across to the Mojave Desert and that extends west to east 68 miles from Tejon Pass to Cajon Pass. It can be said that the mountains act as both hero and villain to the Southland's millions: they gather moisture from Pacific storms, but at the same time they increase urban air pollution by locking in air masses.

Geologists tell us that the range is a massive block of the earth's crust, separated from the surrounding landscape by a network of major faults—the San Andreas Fault on the north, the San Gabriel and Sierra Madre Faults on the south, and the Soledad Fault on the west. The great block itself, in turn, is fractured by numerous subsidiary faults. The result is an extremely uneven surface. Eons of erosive stream action have cut deep V-shaped canyons, further accentuating the unevenness. The surface rocks are fractured and intermixed in great confusion, forming a heterogeneous mixture of crystalline limestone, schists, and quartzites, which have been invaded by intrusive granites and other igneous rocks, all forming a most complicated mass.

Covering about 80% of this wrinkled mountain mass is a thick blanket of stiff, thorny shrubs and dwarf trees collectively called chaparral: chamise, scrub oak, yucca, wild lilac, mountain mahogany, laurel, snowbrush (whitethorn), chinquapin, and that unpopular champion of all rigidity, manzanita. This elfin forest, where it has not recently been burned off—for it grows quickly back—fastens securely to hillsides, seizing every square foot not preempted by timber or crag or rockfield. It swarms over hot, exposed slopes whose conditions it alone can endure, spreading until it forms an almost impenetrable collar between the foothills and the high pine country.

Chaparral has been damned as too low to give shade, too high to see over, and too thick to go through. Anyone so foolish as to venture off road or trail and crawl through this brushy maze will soon come to believe that there is a personal hostility in the unyielding branches and scratchy leaves.

A different experience awaits those who consider this forest as a friend to visit, not as an enemy to thrash through. In bloom, much of the chaparral is sprinkled with colorful flowers. And what is more pleasing to the nature lover than ceanothus blooming into misty blue or white, giving forth its sweet aroma after a spring rain? Or checkerspot butterflies collecting nectar from yerba santa? Chaparral is also valuable as a soil cover; where it has been burned off, rain rushes down the hillsides, causing severe erosion on the slopes and flooding in the canyons.

Below the chaparral belt, in the canyons, a luxuriant cover of sycamore, live oak, alder, and bay trees shields sparkling streams from the sun's glare. Above the chaparral, and sometimes as enclaves within it, is a cool, stately world of conifers: first big-cone Douglas-firs, and then—progressively higher—Coulter and ponderosa pines, Jeffrey pines, incense cedars, sugar pines, white firs, and lodgepole pines. On the highest ridges, subalpine conditions reign, and gnarled limber pines live a marginal existence among windswept crags.

The wildlife of the San Gabriel Mountains is timid—as well it should be. Humans have preempted most of the range, crowding out animals that once roamed in abundance. Some species are gone completely: no longer does the giant California condor soar overhead (although the occasional straggler sometimes wanders over from Ventura County), nor the mammoth grizzly bear prowl the forest. Both disappeared from here shortly after the turn of the 20th century. Often seen in the San Gabriels and in nearby foothill communities is the black bear; naturalists estimate their number to be anywhere from 250 to 300. All of the bears in the range are descendants of an initial population of 11 troublemakers deported from Yosemite National Park in 1933. In the remote recesses of the range, an estimated 250 Nelson bighorn sheep scratch out a living, and the population has suffered a steep decline in the past few decades; experts are unsure of the exact causes. You must walk far from the highway to see these noble animals, deep into the rugged San Gabriel and Cucamonga Wildernesses or high up on the stony battlements of Iron Mountain.

The most abundant large mammal in the San Gabriels is the California mule deer, usually yellow-brown in summer, gray in winter, its many-pronged antlers growing to considerable size. Preying on the deer are a number of mountain lions, perhaps 40 or 50 in the whole range. In recent years, sightings of these agile beasts have increased, and several well-publicized attacks have occurred. Although the odds of an encounter are slight, hikers should be vigilant, and children should never be left unattended. Smaller mammals include the bobcat, ring-tailed cat, gray fox, weasel, and skunk, along with a host of squirrels and chipmunks. The region's most common creature considered sometimes dangerous to humans is the western rattlesnake, abundant below 6,000 feet, and sometimes seen up to 8,000 feet. However, most rattlers are not very aggressive and usually won't bother you unless you bother them by picking them up or stepping on them.

Geographically, the San Gabriels are for most of their length made up of two roughly parallel ranges. The northern, inland range is the longer and loftier, extending from Mount Gleason and Mount Pacifico eastward past the 8,000-foot and 9,000-foot summits of Waterman, Williamson, Islip, Hawkins, Throop, and Baden-Powell, and climaxing near its eastern end in the only summit over 10,000 feet—Mount San Antonio (Old Baldy) and its cluster of satellite peaks. The southern, or front, range, though neither as long nor as high, is equally rugged. Two of its summits—Strawberry and San Gabriel—exceed 6,000 feet, and 10 others exceed 5,000 feet. Below

Mountain lion near Chilao

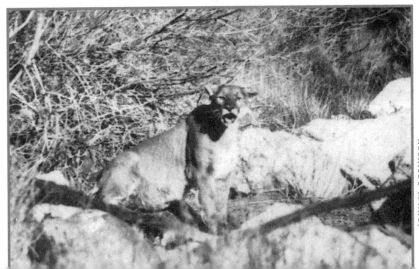

the peaks is a complex of deep, shaded canyons, extending well up into the higher parts of the range. The range's major watershed is the San Gabriel River, whose three main forks and countless tributaries drain fully 20% of the mountain precipitation. Other important watersheds are Pacoima, Little Tujunga, Big Tujunga, Arroyo Seco, Santa Anita, San Antonio, and Lytle Creek Canyons on the south slope of the range, and Little Rock and Big Rock Creeks on the north.

Finally, there is the Liebre Mountain–Sawmill Mountain–Sierra Pelona country to the northwest of the San Gabriels proper, beyond the great wind gap of Soledad Canyon. Geographers disagree on whether this gentle mountain region of long, whale-backed ridges and shallow canyons belongs to the San Gabriels, the Tehachapis, or neither. But it is part of Angeles National Forest and it is good hiking country, so it is included here.

No other mountain range in California is so accessible to so many people for so little effort—and year-round. When winter's white mantle closes off the high country, the woodsy canyons and green-velvet foothills become refreshing, delightful, and inviting. And then, in turn, when summer's sweltering dryness invades canyon and foothill, the high mountains once again beckon. For this all-season aspect, and for the San Gabriels themselves— ageless, rock-ribbed, and aromatic with the restoring scents of forest and chaparral—shall we ever be thankful.

Humans in the San Gabriels

HUMANS HAVE ENTERED the San Gabriels in almost every conceivable manner. We have come into the mountains for a multitude of reasons. And we have come in great numbers. Few mountain ranges anywhere have been so viewed, swarmed over, dug into, and built upon by the human species.

What draws us to the mountains? Is it curiosity? The promise of adventure? The excitement of hunting and fishing? The chance of a better livelihood? The quest for mineral wealth? The longing to redeem and revitalize oneself, away from the hustle of urban life? The need for something spiritual or ego-satisfying? The long pageant of humans in the San Gabriels reveals all these motives, along with some that are not so readily identified. The fascination of the canyons, the ridges, the peaks, and the little flats that lie deep in the mountains has attracted human visitors since humans first made their home in Southern California. People have come to the mountains, have seen, have lingered, and in many cases have remained for life.

One might suppose that the San Gabriels would be worn out (ecologically) by all this human activity. Some parts are, particularly in the front range. Fortunately, though, there are other areas where human impact has been minimal, where nature still rules—thanks to the protective efforts of a handful of people who, for a variety of reasons ranging from enlightened self-interest to aesthetic values, have fought to save the mountains and the forests for the benefit of all. Humankind is not totally shortsighted, although we often appear to be.

The first humans in the San Gabriels were Shoshone Indian peoples— Tongva in the southern foothills and Serranos in the eastern and northern high country. Other tribal groups in the Liebre–Sawmill–Sierra Pelona country were the Alliklik and Kitanemuk peoples, also Shoshonean. Though their homes were generally below the mountains, these peoples depended heavily on the San Gabriel range. The mountains supplied them with food, water, and materials for building and hunting. For food, they hunted deer and rabbits and gathered acorns and pine nuts. They took water from the streams that gushed down from great heights. Chaparral was an abundant source of many necessities. Manzanita berries were pressed for cider, and the leaves were smoked. Greasewood provided arrow shafts for hunting. Yucca fibers were used to make nets and ropes.

To obtain these materials, and to visit and trade with other peoples across the range, Native Americans made the first footpaths into the mountains. According to Will Thrall, foremost collector of San Gabriel Mountains history, who personally searched out these ancient routes at a time when they could still be followed, the main Shoshone trail across the range ascended Millard Canyon, traversed behind Mount Lowe to Red Box Saddle, descended the West Fork San Gabriel River to Valley Forge Canyon, climbed up that canyon to Barley Flats, went down and across the head of Big Tujunga Canyon and up to Pine (Charlton) Flat, and continued to the west end of Chilao. Here, the trail forked. One branch followed the high country northeast to Buckhorn and then went down the South Fork of Little Rock Creek to the desert. The other branch dropped northwest into upper Alder

Creek. It then ascended Indian Ridge (where traces of the old footpath can still be seen) to Sheep Camp Spring on the west slope of Mount Pacifico and dropped down Santiago Canyon to Little Rock Creek and along it to the desert. Another cross-range trail ascended the North Fork San Gabriel River, climbed over Windy Gap, and descended the South Fork of Big Rock Creek to the desert. For perhaps two or three centuries before the arrival of the white settlers, these and many shorter canyon trails were trod by hundreds of Native Americans every year.

The arrival of the Spaniards changed life in the pleasant valleys below the mountains forever. In 1771, along the grassy banks of the Rio Hondo, Mission San Gabriel Arcángel was founded, and soon thereafter, the Gabrielinos were forcibly incorporated into the mission community. Mission San Fernando Rey de España, founded in 1797, became the home of the less-numerous Fernandeños. At the height of mission activity—around 1800—these two outposts of the cross numbered some 2,000 Native Americans in their widespread flocks. The San Gabriel Mountains became a haven for refugees fleeing abusive mission life.

Several decades later came the era of the great ranchos, bringing a pastoral way of life to the valleys. These spacious cattle ranches that spread out below the south slopes of the range bore the familiar names of San Fernando, Tujunga, La Cañada, San Pascual, Santa Anita, Azusa de Duarte, and San Jose.

The Spanish and Mexican Californios used the mountains very little except as a source of water. When there were buildings to be constructed, woodcutters sometimes took timber from the lower canyons. Vaqueros did some hunting in the canyons and foothills. Grizzly bears, numerous in the range then, were stalked and captured, and then dragged to the bull ring in the Pueblo of Los Angeles to be sacrificed in brutal bear-bull contests.

There is no evidence that the Spaniards ever penetrated the heart of the mountains, although they certainly explored the fringes. Gaspar de Portolá and Pedro Fages, on their epic journey northward in 1769, toiled through the narrow canyon of San Fernando Pass and found "high, barren hills, very difficult for beasts of burden" before dropping into pleasant Newhall Valley. On another path-finding trip in 1772, Fages crossed the eastern end of the range in the vicinity of Cajon Pass and continued northwest below the northern ramparts of the mountains, discovering the Joshua trees. Fray Francisco Garcés, the missionary/explorer/martyr, explored both sides of the range in 1776. Fray José María Zalvidea almost circled what is now Angeles National Forest in 1806.

It was the Spaniards who gave the mountains their name—two names, in fact, that have existed side by side until relatively recent years. In 1776 Garcés referred to the range as Sierra de San Gabriel, borrowing the name of the nearby mission, and this name was used in Spanish records frequently in ensuing years. But the mission padres usually referred to the range as Sierra Madre ("mother range"). Both *San Gabriel* and *Sierra Madre* were in common usage until 1927 when the U.S. Board on Geographic Names finally ruled in favor of the former. Today *San Gabriel Mountains* is almost universally accepted.

With the coming of the Anglos—from the 1840s onward—the San Gabriels began to receive more attention. Prospectors, hunters, bandits, homesteaders, and squatters were pioneers in unveiling the secrets of the mountains. These hardy individuals first entered the wooded canyons, and then forged their way over the ridges and into the hidden heart of the range—terrain the rancheros had scorned.

Stories of gold in the San Gabriels go back as far as the 1770s, but not until 1842, when Francisco Lopez discovered gold clinging to the roots of a cluster of wild onions in Placerita Canyon, near present-day Newhall, was there what might be called a gold rush. The San Fernando Placers, as the discovery was called, were worked on and off for about a decade, until strikes elsewhere drew the miners away. By far, the largest gold strike in the San Gabriels occurred on the East Fork San Gabriel River. The precious metal was discovered in the canyon gravels in 1854, and for the next seven years the East Fork was the scene of frenzied activity, with an estimated $2 million in gold being recovered (worth about $60 million in 2020 dollars). A smaller strike occurred in Big Santa Anita Canyon about the same time. During the next half century, prospectors rushed into the mountains at every rumor of bonanza, tearing up hillsides in their frantic search for wealth.

Bandits, including Jack Powers, Salomon Pico, Juan Flores, and the legendary Tiburcio Vásquez, turned to the San Gabriels for refuge. They drove stolen cattle and horses up the canyons and pastured them in backcountry flats. Using the faint network of old Native American trails, these outlaws established isolated hideouts deep in the mountains.

The pioneer trail builder in the San Gabriels was Benjamin Wilson, who in 1864 reworked an old Native American path up Little Santa Anita Canyon to the top of the mountain that now bears his name. During the next three decades, trails were blazed up all the major canyons of the front range, some of them continuing over the ridges and into the backcountry. In increasing numbers, homesteaders and squatters followed these trails and found favorite spots on which to build their cabins. The names of many of these early mountain men have endured to the present, attached to canyons, camps, and peaks—Wilson, Millard, Henninger, Newcomb, Chantry, Vincent, Islip, and Dawson, among others.

Almost all of these pioneers came into the mountains for utilitarian reasons—to mine gold, to cut timber, to find refuge, to pasture livestock, or to establish a home. Around 1885 a new reason for going to the mountains arose—recreation. Great numbers of San Gabriel Valley residents journeyed to Mount Wilson on weekends and holidays to enjoy the cool mountain air and take in the fabulous panorama. (This was before air pollution muddled Southland skies.) Hunters entered the range seeking big game, which was plentiful in the San Gabriels until around the turn of the 20th century. Grizzly bears, deer, mountain sheep, and mountain lions were stalked by bands of thrill-seeking hunters who penetrated far into the mountains. Sportsmen packed in for a week's fishing on the trout-filled West Fork San Gabriel River. For the less energetic, there were Sunday afternoon picnics in such woodsy haunts as Millard and Eaton Canyons.

Other people entered the mountains for a different reason: exploitation. Most Americans of that day assumed that our natural resources were inexhaustible and therefore did not need to be conserved. Lumber was needed to fuel Southern California's great boom of the 1880s; why not use the timber close at hand? Indiscriminate cutting of forest trees appeared imminent. Furthermore, the value of chaparral for the mountain watershed was little understood. Brush fires, some deliberately set by cattlemen to clear land for grazing, raged across the mountains until extinguished by rain. Fortunately, some farsighted residents in Los Angeles and the San Gabriel Valley became alarmed at this exploitation and devastation of the local mountains, and they began working to preserve the lands.

One of these was Abbot Kinney, a rancher, botanist, and land developer who lived at his Kinneloa Ranch above Altadena. Kinney is best remembered as the creator of Venice, the Southern California beach town that once had canals for streets, but it was as chairman of California's first Board of Forestry that he did his most important work. In the first report of the Board of Forestry to Governor George Stoneman in 1886, Kinney urged "intelligent supervision of the forest land and brush lands of California, with a view to their preservation." This California movement for forest conservation, sparked by Kinney and others, soon became part of a national movement. John Muir, using his eloquence in a series of magazine articles urging forest protection, was the leading spokesman.

Congress finally responded by passing the Forest Reserve Act of 1891, granting the president the authority "to set apart and reserve . . . any part of the public lands wholly or in part covered with timber or undergrowth." As a result of this act and strong pressure from Southern California civic leaders, President Benjamin Harrison signed the bill establishing the San Gabriel Timberland Reserve on December 20, 1892. This was the first forest reserve in California and the second in the United States. (The first was the Yellowstone Park Timberland Reserve in Wyoming, established by presidential proclamation

Clouds over southeast ridge of Mount Wilson (see Hike 39)

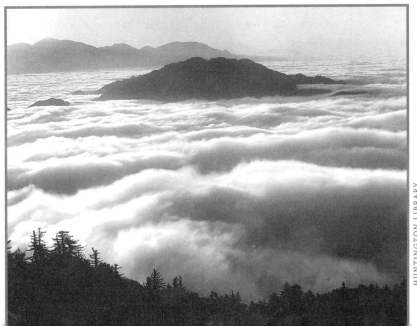

HUNTINGTON LIBRARY

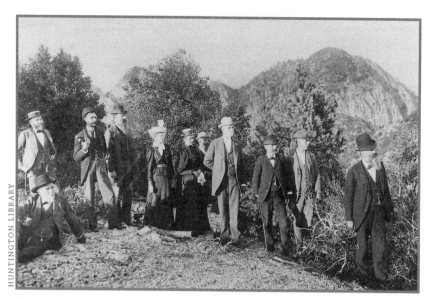

Thaddeus S. C. Lowe (center) and party on Mount Lowe (1892)

on September 16, 1891.) The designation was at first rather ineffectual; for one thing, forest rangers were not assigned until 1898. But gradually the San Gabriel Timberland Reserve was brought under efficient forest management and protection. In 1907 the name was changed to San Gabriel National Forest, and the following year it became what we know today—Angeles National Forest. A succession of capable supervisors—Everett Thomas, Theodore Lukens, Rush Charlton, William Mendenhall, Sim Jarvi, William Dresser, and Paul Sweetland—got the national forest off to an excellent start.

Worldwide fame came to the San Gabriels in the 1890s with construction of the Mount Lowe Scenic Railway, considered one of the engineering wonders of its time. This breathtaking cable incline and trolley ride—along with associated hotels in Rubio Canyon, atop Echo Mountain, and on the slopes of Mount Lowe—was the brainchild of inventor Thaddeus S. C. Lowe and engineer David Macpherson. The famed mountain railway-resort complex attracted more than 3 million visitors during its 43 years of operation.

The human quest for scientific knowledge played its part in the story of the mountains too. In the days before city lights and air pollution interfered with sky viewing, Mount Wilson's broad summit was ideal for astronomical observation. The first telescope on Mount Wilson was the 13-incher of

Harvard University Observatory, placed on the summit in 1889 (but removed the following year). The year 1904 saw the beginning of the Carnegie Institute's famed Mount Wilson Observatory, one of the 20th century's great scientific ventures. Largely through the initiative and enthusiasm of astronomer George Ellery Hale, several of the world's greatest telescopes were erected on the mountaintop, the most important being the 60-inch reflector (1908), the 150-foot solar tower telescope (1912), and the 100-inch Hooker reflector (1917), the latter the world's largest optical telescope for 31 years.

Before highways crisscrossed the San Gabriels, the mountains were the delight of hikers. Historians call the period from about 1895 to 1938 the Great Hiking Era. Multitudes of lowland residents enjoyed their weekends and holidays rambling over the range. Trails that today are almost deserted vibrated with the busy tramp of boots. The mountains were a local frontier for exploration and a challenge to the hardy. For some, hiking was simply a favorite sport; for others, it was almost a religion. Trail resorts sprang up to offer hospitality, food, and lodging to hikers. Such places as Switzer's, Opid's, Colby's, Loomis's, Sturtevant's, and Roberts's were visited by thousands every season.

A strange combination of disasters and "progress" brought the Great Hiking Era to a close. The disasters were a series of fires and consequent floods, the great destructive torrent of March 1938 being the final blow. Overnight, miles of canyon trails were obliterated. "Progress" took the form of the Angeles Crest Highway, begun in 1929. Relentlessly, the great asphalt thoroughfare snaked its way into the heart of the mountains, reaching Red Box in 1934, Charlton Flat in 1937, and Chilao a year later. By 1941 it had inched its way across Cloudburst Summit and reached that most isolated of backcountry haunts, Buckhorn. Places that once required a day or two of strenuous hiking were now accessible in an hour of driving. One by one, the old trail resorts succumbed. As one old-timer sadly reflected, "Only people who hike for the love of hiking use these trails now." The Angeles Crest Highway, more than anything else, changed the pattern of our use of the San Gabriels.

In recent years, great numbers of people have visited the San Gabriels, the vast majority by automobile, and visitation is increasing. Each year there are an estimated 3.5 million visits to the Angeles National Forest, making the Angeles one of the most heavily used national forests in the United States.

As use has increased, the wilderness aspect of the mountains has come under pressure. Other than the designated wilderness areas and a few other

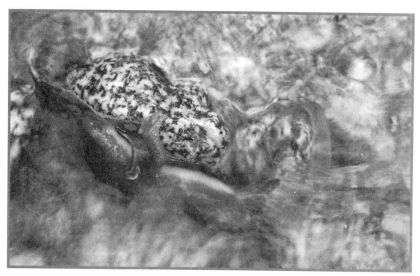

California newt

small, isolated regions, the San Gabriels have in recent years become not much more than a king-size backyard playground for Los Angeles County. Some say that this is as it should be, but recent ecological studies have tended to show that wilderness undisturbed by humans plays a vital part in nature's delicate balance among living things.

Angeles National Forest today encompasses 700,176 acres. Within this mountain area are more than 1,000 miles of roads, 548 miles of riding and hiking trails, 36 public campgrounds, 25 picnic areas, 463 summer residences, five wilderness areas, and five winter sports areas.

The future of the San Gabriels—as well as all other mountain ranges—rests with the population that lives nearby. In the words of mountain historian Charles Clark Vernon, "They are truly a gift to the people." What the people will do with this gift of nature remains to be seen.

THE STATION AND BOBCAT FIRES

THE SAN GABRIEL MOUNTAINS are being transformed by fire during our lifetime. The 2009 Station Fire was the largest fire in the San Gabriel Mountains, consuming more than 160,000 acres encompassing much of the western third of the range. The fire was started by an arsonist and killed two firefighters. The burn zone was closed to public entry for many years

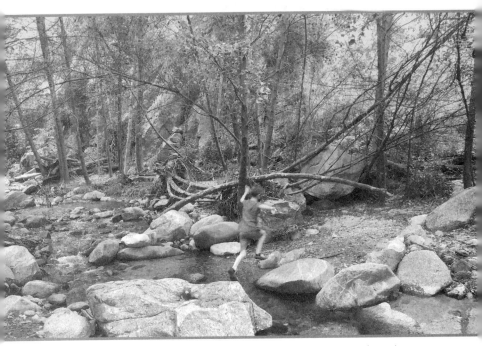

Rock-hopping on the Arroyo Seco near Teddy's Outpost (see Hike 11)

until enough vegetation took root to discourage illegal off-road drivers, and it took nearly a decade to reopen all trails. The Santa Clara Divide Road to Messenger Flats remains closed at the time of this writing.

As this book is going into production in November 2020, the Bobcat Fire is still smoldering after sweeping across 115,796 acres and damaging or destroying more than 100 homes. It started near Cogswell Dam on the West Fork San Gabriel River during intensely hot and dry conditions. The cause is still under investigation, but Southern California Edison reported an equipment malfunction nearby around the time smoke was first observed. The fire burned most of the central part of the range between the Station Fire boundary and Highway 39. The U.S. Forest Service issued a closure order through at least April 1, 2022, closing the burn area as well as some nearby unburned trails, impacting a third of the hikes in this book. These hikes are flagged with a note at the beginning of the hike profile and in the chart on page xiii. The extent of trail damage is not yet fully known. I surveyed the San Gabriel Mountains from the air in October 2020 and have commented in the note about whether obvious damage was visible. The most severe burns were in the West Fork San Gabriel River, Bear Creek, Big Santa Anita Canyon, and Monrovia Canyon watersheds and along the north slopes near Devil's Punchbowl. The forest along the Angeles Crest between Cloudburst Summit and Dawson Saddle experienced patchy burns. Based on the aftermath of the Station Fire, some trails may take years to reopen. *Caution:* Never take a rest break or camp near burned trees, which might blow down on you.

These fires may permanently change the ecology of the San Gabriel Mountains. Some of the pine and fir forests may be replaced by chaparral, and some of the lower chaparral belts may be replaced with desert scrub. We are witnessing the impact of climate change on our beloved mountains.

Hiking Hints

TRAVELING A MOUNTAIN TRAIL, away from centers of civilization, is a unique experience in Southern California living. It brings intimate association with nature—communion with the earth, the forest, the chaparral, the wildlife, and the clear sky. A great responsibility accompanies this experience: the obligation to keep the mountains as you found them. Being considerate of the wilderness rights of others will make the mountain adventures of those who follow equally rewarding.

As a mountain visitor, you should become familiar with the rules of wilderness courtesy, outlined below.

TRAILS

NEVER CUT SWITCHBACKS. This practice breaks down trails and hastens erosion. Take care not to dislodge rocks that might fall on hikers below you. Improve and preserve trails by clearing away loose rocks (carefully) and removing branches. Report any trail damage and broken or misplaced signs to a ranger.

OFF TRAIL

RESTRAIN THE IMPULSE to blaze trees or to build cairns where not essential. Let the next hikers find their way as you did.

MOUNTAIN BIKES

MOUNTAIN BIKERS NEED to respect the rights and the safety of hikers and horseback riders and should follow sound conservation practices. Yield right-of-way to other trail users. Control your speed. Stay off muddy trails, and do not shortcut switchbacks. Mountain biking is permissible on most forest trails but is prohibited in wilderness areas and on the Pacific Crest Trail.

CAMPGROUNDS

SPREAD YOUR GEAR in an area that has already been cleared, and build your fire in a campground stove. Don't build hard-to-eradicate ramparts of rock for fireplaces or windbreaks. Rig tents and tarps with line tied to rocks or trees; never put nails in trees. For your campfire, use fallen wood only; do not cut standing trees or break off branches. Open campfires are allowed only in fire rings at established campgrounds; fires are prohibited at wilderness campsites. Use the campground latrine. Place your litter in the litter can or carry it out. Leave the campground cleaner than you found it.

FIRE

FIRE IS THE GREATEST DANGER in the Southern California mountains; act accordingly. Do not make campfires outside of designated campgrounds and picnic areas. Extingish the campfire with water before leaving it unattended; then stir, mix, and feel the ashes to ensure no warm spots remain. To use a camp stove outside a developed recreation area, you must obtain a free California Campfire Permit from a U.S. Forest Service office or online at ready forwildfire.org/permits/campfire-permit.

During times of high danger, campfires and camp stoves are prohibited even in campgrounds. Smoking is permitted only in campgrounds, places of habitation, and vehicles. Report a mountain fire immediately to the National Interagency Fire Center (208-387-5512) or 911.

LITTER

ALONG THE TRAIL, place candy wrappers, drink bottles, orange peels, and so on in your pocket or pack for later disposal; throw nothing on the trail.

Bury human waste and toilet paper at least 6 inches deep and at least 200 feet from trails, water, and campsites. Pick up litter you find along the trail or in camp. More than almost anything else, litter detracts from the wilderness scene. Remember, you can take it with you.

NOISE

BOISTEROUS CONDUCT is out of harmony in a wilderness experience. Be a considerate hiker and camper; don't ruin others' enjoyment of the mountains with excess noise.

HIKER ETHICS

HUMAN LIFE AND WELL-BEING take precedence over most everything else—in the mountains as elsewhere. If a hiker or camper is in trouble, help in any way you can. Give comfort or first aid, and then hurry to a ranger station for help.

Maps

IT IS IMPORTANT to know where you are in relation to roads, campgrounds, landmarks, and so on, and to have a general understanding of the lay of the land. For this orientation there is no substitute for a good map. Unless your trip is short and over a well-marked route, you should carry a map.

Besides the shaded-relief trail map that accompanies this book, there are several other types of maps that will give you the picture you need of the San Gabriel Mountains. Each type has its advantages and disadvantages.

This book is accompanied by the free eTrails app for iOS users, available through the Apple App Store. eTrails contains high-quality maps and waypoints for these trips, as well as for the Pacific Crest Trail and several of the author's other guidebooks; it also provides driving directions from your present position to the trailheads. In the app, go to the Menu tab, select "ToA10e," and then pick the hike that interests you. The GPS tracks and waypoints for most of the trips in this book can also be downloaded directly from eTrails.net. You can use them with Gaia or other apps on your mobile device or computer, or copy them onto a handheld GPS unit.

Previous editions of this book recommended the U.S. Geological Survey (USGS) topographic maps and the U.S. Forest Service recreation maps. Unfortunately, the USGS maps have not kept up with trail changes, and the Forest Service maps aren't much more detailed than the trail map accompanying this book.

Nowadays, Tom Harrison makes the most accurate and cost-effective paper maps for this region. His *Angeles Front Country* map covers the western end of the range, and his *Angeles High Country* map covers the eastern end. They are also available for the Avenza Maps app on iOS and Android devices, where they have the extra benefit of showing your position overlaying the map and the drawback of leaving you stranded if your battery runs out. Visit tomharrisonmaps.com to buy the electronic version.

The National Geographic Trails Illustrated *Angeles National Forest* map covers the entire range, including the area around Liebre Mountain and Sierra Pelona that is not on the Tom Harrison map. Unfortunately, this map has many errors, but it is still useful for casual hiking.

Both Tom Harrison and Trails Illustrated waterproof maps are available at most ranger stations, from REI and other bookstores and outdoor stores, and from many online sellers.

For cross-country navigation, you may want a topographic map showing finer detail over a smaller area. CalTopo.com has topographic maps with fairly accurate trail information that you can examine and print for free.

Using This Book

THE HIKING TRIPS in this guide are arranged by geographical area, generally west to east. Information about each trip is divided into three parts: Trip, Features, and Description.

The **Trip** section gives vital statistics: where the hike starts and ends; the walking mileage and elevation gain or loss; a rating of easy, moderate, or strenuous; the best time of year to make the trip; and the appropriate map or maps. Trips more than 5 miles long are generally rounded to the nearest mile.

The **Features** section tells something of what you will see on the trip and gives information on the natural and human history of the area. It also contains suggestions for the particular trip, such as "wear lug-soled boots" or "bring fishing rod."

The **Description** section details driving and hiking routes. The driving directions are kept to the necessary minimum, while the walking route is described in detail. Also, hiking options that a trip presents are described.

The hikes have been graded as easy, moderate, or strenuous. An easy trip is usually 4 miles or less in horizontal distance, with less than a 500-foot elevation gain—suitable for beginners and children. A moderate trip—including the majority here—is a 5- to 10-mile hike, usually with less than a 2,500-foot elevation difference. You should be in fair physical condition for these, and children under age 12 might find the going difficult. Strenuous trips are all-day rambles involving many miles of hiking and much elevation gain and loss; they are only for those in top physical condition and with hiking experience. The most important criteria for grading a trip were mileage covered, elevation gain and loss, and condition of the trail. Of less significance were accessibility of terrain, availability of water, exposure to sun, and ground cover. Obviously, some of the latter criteria depend on the weather and the time of year: a 3-mile hike over open chaparral slopes can be miserable under the hot August sun but delightful in January's cool breeze and cloudiness.

A season recommendation is also included for each trip. This classification is particularly important in the lower, south-facing parts of the range, where summer and fall bring fire danger.

Campfires are permitted only in fire rings in designated campgrounds and picnic areas. Gas-type portable stoves may be used if you obtain a California campfire permit—available at any ranger station or visitor center. In conditions of extreme fire danger, the forest may be closed to entry off of major highways. In recent years a series of disastrous infernos have taken a heavy toll, both in property damage and in the cost required to fight the fires.

This edition adds GPS waypoints for the trailhead and destination of each hike and occasionally for key points along the way (especially for trips with cross-country travel). Distances along the route are reported to the nearest 0.1 mile. Be aware that two GPS units, even carried by the same person on the same day, can report substantially different distances. Quality of satellite reception and filtering of noise in the GPS software substantially affect the readings, so don't rely on exact distances.

WILDERNESS PERMITS

THERE ARE FIVE WILDERNESS AREAS in the San Gabriels: Cucamonga, Sheep Mountain, San Gabriel, Pleasant View Ridge, and Magic Mountain. A free permit is required for entry into the Cucamonga Wilderness east of Icehouse Saddle and for entry into the Sheep Mountain Wilderness from the East Fork trailhead only.

NATIONAL FOREST ADVENTURE PASS REQUIREMENT

YOU MUST DISPLAY a National Forest Adventure Pass in your parked vehicle at trailheads providing picnic tables and toilet facilities in the national forests of Southern California. Adventure Passes cost $30 for an annual pass, $5 for a day pass, or $80 for the annual America the Beautiful Pass that also covers national parks; they can be purchased at ranger stations, visitor centers, and many business establishments in or near the mountains. According to the *Fragosa v. Moore* settlement agreement of 2016, the U.S. Forest Service is required to allow free roadside parking within 0.5 mile of the trailhead for visitors who are not using the picnic or toilet facilities. As of this writing, the Forest Service has generally not updated signage or advertised such free parking.

■ 100 Hikes in ■
the San Gabriel
Mountains

▪ Hike 1 LIEBRE MOUNTAIN 🥾 🐕 🚶

HIKE LENGTH 7 miles out-and-back; 1,700' elevation gain

DIFFICULTY Moderate

SEASON All year

MAP Trails Illustrated *Angeles National Forest*

PERMIT N/A

▪ FEATURES

The long whaleback of Liebre Mountain sprawls at the northwest corner of Angeles National Forest, where the Coast Ranges, the Tehachapis, and the San Gabriels all meld together in a wrinkled jumble. From Liebre's broad summit, you look north across golden-brown Antelope Valley to the Tehachapis, curving from west to northeast in a great arc; and if the day is clear, the southern ramparts of the Sierra Nevada are visible on the distant skyline. Southward, you peer into the gentle ridge-and-canyon country of the Cienega and Fish

Canyon watersheds. The mountain itself is named for the 1846 Mexican land grant Rancho La Liebre; *liebre* is Spanish for "rabbit."

This is delightful mountain country, especially in spring, when snow patches linger on north slopes, the California black oak is clothing itself with reddish leaves, and aromatic white sage is blooming in the foothills. This is the home of the gray pine, a hardy dweller on semiarid slopes, easily identifiable by its gray-green needles, large cones (second in size only to the Coulter pine), and multiforked trunk. Also on the mountainside are big-cone

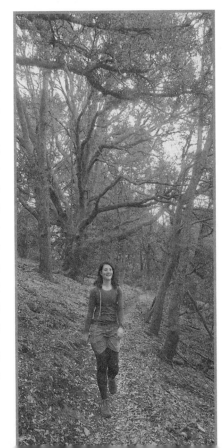

*Beneath the oaks on
Liebre Mountain*

Douglas-firs and some rather large scrub oaks. Occasional junipers and piñon pines bear testimony to the blending of mountain and desert here.

This trip follows the historic old Horse Trail, now part of the Pacific Crest Trail but once used to drive horses from the Tejon Ranch to Los Angeles, steeply up the forested north slope of Liebre Mountain from Horse Trail Flat to the summit. Do it in leisurely fashion to fully appreciate the desert view and the unique combination of forest trees and chaparral. It's a long drive from Los Angeles, but the mountainside is remote, peaceful, and beautiful—well worth the effort.

The summit of Liebre Mountain was near the western perimeter of the 31,089-acre 2020 Lake Fire.

■ DESCRIPTION

From I-5 north of Santa Clarita, take Exit 198A to go east on Highway 138. Go 4 miles, then turn right on the Old Ridge Route (County Road N2). In 2.2 miles turn left onto Pine Canyon Road (also CR N2). In 4.3 miles, at a crest of a hill just beyond mile marker 13.6, turn right (south) on a rutted dirt road. Follow the road 0.1 mile to its end at the Pacific Crest Trail (GPS N34° 44.306' W118° 39.357'). If the road is washed out and your vehicle has low clearance, consider parking on the shoulder of Pine Canyon Road instead.

At the upper edge of the parking area is the Pacific Crest Trail (PCT), the southbound section climbing west, the northbound dropping southeast. Take the southbound PCT, which ascends the mountainside. (If you start descending, you're on the wrong trail segment.) You switchback up through live oaks and gray pines, with far-ranging views over Antelope Valley to the Tehachapis. After 2.0 miles you pass Horse Camp to your right. A table and fire ring are here, but there's no water. (Water can be found seasonally in Horse Camp Canyon via a short use trail from the camp.) You continue switchbacking upward, under a cool canopy of pines and oaks. Near the top, your trail becomes an old jeep track. About 60 yards before you reach the crest and a junction with Forest Road 7N23, turn right and scramble to the small rock cairn that marks the 5,760-foot summit of Liebre Mountain (GPS N34° 42.755' W118° 39.255'). Beware of the foxtail barley around the summit, as it has barbs that catch in your socks or could injure a dog's eyes. Return the way you came.

VARIATION With a 5-mile car or bicycle shuttle, you can follow the Liebre hogback west and drop down to the Old Ridge Route at the former site of the historic Sandberg Inn, 0.5 mile south of the Pine Canyon turnoff. You can follow either the easy Liebre Mountain Truck Trail or the more scenic Golden Eagle Trail, an abandoned segment of the PCT that crisscrosses the dirt road. This route is 10 miles.

■ Hike 2 FISH CANYON NARROWS 🡕 🐐 ◉ 🚶

> **HIKE LENGTH** 10 miles out-and-back; 800' elevation gain
>
> **DIFFICULTY** Moderate
>
> **SEASON** All year
>
> **MAP** Trails Illustrated *Angeles National Forest*
>
> **PERMIT** N/A

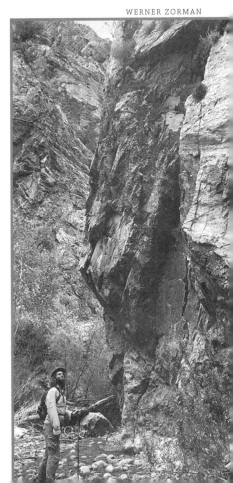

WERNER ZORMAN

■ FEATURES

The long, shallow, meandering canyons in the northwest corner of the Angeles National Forest are almost all laden with asphalt ribbon. One exception, and perhaps the most scenic canyon of them all, is Fish Canyon, which runs south from Sawmill Mountain and then southwest into the Castaic Creek drainage.

Fish Canyon offers the best hiking in this part of the Angeles. A year-round stream descends its length, shaded most of the way by clusters of oaks, sycamores, alders, and willows. For the most part, the canyon is open and gently sloped—except the 0.5-mile stretch of Fish Canyon Narrows,

Admiring Fish Canyon Narrows
above Pianobox

a slot through the mountain sometimes only a few yards wide. Abrupt, towering sidewalls of colorful rock make these narrows the most spectacular in the range—a Grand Canyon in miniature.

This pleasant, almost level streamside trip ascends Fish Canyon from Castaic Creek; follows a dirt road to Cienega Campground and then trail onto the Pianobox, an old mining prospect; and then passes through the scenic narrows to Rogers Trail Camp. Be sure to wear stout waterproof boots for the many stream crossings. Wear bright colors in October, when hunters frequent the area.

■ DESCRIPTION

From I-5 north of Castaic, take Exit 183 east on Templin Highway. In 4.3 miles, find a parking spot on the shoulder before a gate that blocks the highway, where a private LADWP road turns right toward Castaic Lake (GPS N34° 36.140' W118° 40.228').

Walk down the paved, gated Templin Highway 0.6 mile and cross Castaic Creek on a bridge. The road turns south, becomes dirt, and soon forks. Follow the left road as it heads north up the canyon along lower Fish Creek. Soon the sidewalls close in and the scenery becomes lusher and greener, as the road—sometimes paved and sometimes dirt—crosses and recrosses Fish Creek several times. After walking 2.9 miles from your car, you come to the abandoned Cienega Campground, located in a grove of oaks on a large flat along the creek.

Shortly beyond Cienega Campground, the canyon forks and this trip turns left onto an unsigned trail leading into Fish Canyon. This is a good place to learn to recognize the difference between poison oak and fake poison oak (*Rhus trilobata*), which grow side by side here. Both have leaves in groups of three, but fake poison oak has smaller leaves with a clublike shape. Proceed 1 mile to an old mining prospect called the Pianobox, where you'll find a pleasant campsite beneath a huge coast live oak. Note that campfires are prohibited in Fish Canyon but camp stoves are normally allowed.

From the Pianobox your trail follows the canyon as it turns northeast, and you abruptly enter the cool and shady narrows. Sheer sidewalls of reddish and yellowish rock make this area a favorite of camera enthusiasts. Crossing and recrossing the stream, you work your way slowly upcanyon. In another mile you reach the oak- and sycamore-shaded bench of Rogers Camp, on the left just before the confluence with Burro Canyon (GPS N34° 38.280' W118° 37.657'). Just across the creek you can see a tunnel bored into solid rock, a relic of mining days. This is a good turnaround point.

VARIATION It may be possible to boulder-hop and bushwhack another 4 miles to the former site of Lion Trail Camp at the confluence with Lion Creek. The Fish Canyon Trail once continued 4.5 miles to Atmore Meadows. Little trace remains, although hikers have reported being able to bushwhack through.

Old maps show other trails in the region, but they have been abandoned for decades and are badly overgrown.

▪ Hike 3 SIERRA PELONA 🥾 🐎

> **HIKE LENGTH** 6 miles out-and-back; 1,300' elevation gain
> **DIFFICULTY** Moderate
> **SEASON** All year
> **MAP** Trails Illustrated *Angeles National Forest*
> **PERMIT** N/A

▪ FEATURES

The Sierra Pelona—bare-topped, wind-buffeted, and lonely—forms a long arc across the northern mountains, separating Mint Canyon from first Bouquet Canyon and then Antelope Valley. Standing athwart the great wind funnel of Soledad Canyon, the crest is often battered by hurricane-force gusts. Sierra Pelona Lookout has recorded velocities of up to 100 miles per hour.

This trip follows the Pacific Crest Trail up from Bouquet Canyon and climbs to the top of Sierra Pelona for far-reaching vistas. Do it in summer, fall, winter, or spring—but not on a windy day.

▪ DESCRIPTION

From the 14 Freeway 6 miles east of Santa Clarita, take Exit 9 for Sand Canyon Road north. In 2.0 miles, turn right onto Sierra Highway; then in 0.3 mile, turn left onto Vasquez Canyon Road. In 3.6 miles, turn right onto Bouquet Canyon Road. In 13.7 miles, park at a turnout on the right (near mile 4.3 according to the mile markers; GPS N34° 35.013' W118° 19.299').

From the parking area, take a short trail that climbs to meet the Pacific Crest Trail (PCT). Turn right and step over a gate intended to deter the dirt bikers who illegally use the trail. At 1.0 mile, reach a switchback on a ridge above a second gate, where the PCT turns east and two lightly used trails wander into the chaparral. The old PCT once went this way toward Big Oak Spring, and cyclists still follow the Five Deer Trail, but these trails are currently partially overgrown with many unsigned junctions, so our trip stays on the new PCT up the ridge. At 1.6 miles, the PCT leaves the ridge near a third gate, but a steep firebreak continues up (you could follow this firebreak to a saddle on the ridge). At 2.3 miles, watch for seasonal, piped Bear Spring above the trail. The chaparral gives way to canyon live oaks as you climb. At 3.0 miles, reach the bare crest of Sierra Pelona (GPS N34° 33.978' W118° 19.356'). Your vista now is impressive, especially if you walk a short distance west along the ridgetop fire road. Southeast, across the broad trench of Soledad Canyon, are the peaks of the main range—Mounts Gleason, Pacifico, Waterman, and Williamson. Northwest are the long hogbacks of Liebre and Sawmill Mountains. And north is the desert—sprawling, sun-bleached, and seemingly endless.

VARIATION An option is to walk 3 miles east along the ridgetop fire road to Mount McDill (5,187') for an even better view. Pass a fire road on the left descending to Bouquet Canyon Road and make the final climb to the double-humped summit of McDill. The first hump has a benchmark called Mint, while the second is the true McDill. Histo-

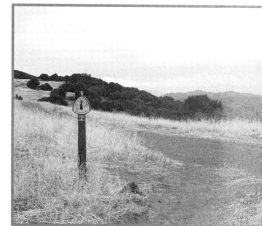

rians speculate that the mountain is named for an early homesteader. The rock outcrops are made of Pelona Schist, a 200-million-year-old metamorphic basement rock that makes up the entire Sierra Pelona ridge and underlies much of the San Gabriel Mountains.

The PCT crosses windswept Sierra Pelona.

■ Hike 4 PLACERITA CANYON PARK ○ 🐴

HIKE LENGTH 7-mile loop; 1,800' elevation gain
DIFFICULTY Moderate
SEASON October–June
MAP Tom Harrison *Angeles Front Country*
PERMIT N/A (free admission)

■ FEATURES

Gentle hills, rounded ridgetops, oak-dotted canyons, and lots of chaparral. This describes the Placerita Canyon country near the western extremity of the main body of the San Gabriels.

Placerita Canyon is etched in history. California's first gold rush occurred here in 1842, six years before John Marshall's famous discovery at Coloma. It began when Francisco Lopez of Rancho San Francisco (near present-day Newhall) grew tired of chasing stray horses and sat down to rest under an oak tree. While resting, Lopez dug up a cluster of wild onions. Clinging to the roots were tiny gold nuggets. The discovery caused much excitement and attracted miners from all over California. These San Fernando Placers, as they become known, produced several hundred thousand dollars in gold before the excitement died down a few years later. Today the gold rush area is preserved as Placerita Canyon State Park. The spot where Lopez is believed to have dug up the gold-bearing onions is known as The Oak of the Golden Dream and is marked with a plaque.

This trip goes up Placerita Canyon, shaded by overarching oaks and sycamores and graced with a trickling creek, to Walker Ranch Campground, and then climbs through chaparral and oaks to Los Pinetos Spring and on to the crest of Los Pinetos Ridge. Here, you are rewarded with far-reaching vistas north across the peaceful Placerita and Sand Canyon country and south across sprawling San Fernando Valley. Then you descend via the Firebreak Ridge–Manzanita Mountain Trail to complete a delightful loop hike.

■ DESCRIPTION

From the 14 Freeway east of Santa Clarita, take Exit 3 and turn right (east) on Placerita Canyon Road. In 1.5 miles, turn right into Placerita Canyon

Natural Area. Continue 0.2 mile to the trailhead parking area by the visitor center (GPS N34° 22.672' W118° 28.058').

Cross the creek and pick up the Canyon Trail, marked by a wooden sign and metal pole, which leads east, on the right side of the creek. The area burned in the 2016 Sand Fire and the canyon washed out, but the trail was rebuilt in 2020. Follow the Canyon Trail 1.9 miles as it winds its way upcanyon, crossing and recrossing the creek (which has water in spring but is usually dry by midsummer) to Walker Ranch Group Campground. Here you reach a trail junction. Turn right onto the Los Pinetos Trail. If you had continued upcanyon, you would have immediately reached a second junction with a spur on the left to Placerita Canyon Road at Walker Ranch and the Waterfall Trail on the right going up Los Pinetos Canyon 0.5 mile to a small cataract, a worthy side trip in the wet season.

The Los Pinetos Trail climbs the chaparral- and oak-coated west slope of Los Pinetos Canyon to Los Pinetos Spring, feeding a nonpotable fire tank nestled in a woodsy recess, 4.1 miles. After a few more switchbacks, reach Santa Clara Divide Road (1N17) at a six-way junction at Wilson Saddle. A short spur trail leads up the hill to picnic benches with outstanding views of the valley.

If the day is hot, you may wish to return the way you came. There is no shade on the remainder of the loop trip. If the day is cool and you wish to continue, turn right (west) and follow the Santa Clara Divide Road uphill until you meet a prominent firebreak leading north, down Firebreak Ridge (4.7 miles). Turn right (north) and follow the firebreak as it descends north then west, over several bumps, to a junction at 6.4 miles with the Manzanita Mountain Trail leading right (north) down to Placerita Canyon State Park. (*Note:* You will see this trail to your right as you descend the last section of the firebreak; there is no sign at the junction, so watch for it carefully.) Descend the trail, passing a short side path on the left that leads 100 yards to the summit of Manzanita Mountain, to reach another junction just above the state park. Go right, passing a water tank, and descend a final 200 feet to the park. Cross Placerita Creek to your car.

■ Hike 5 WHITNEY CANYON ↗ ⊼ 👤 ☀

HIKE LENGTH 3.4 miles out-and-back; 300' elevation gain
DIFFICULTY Easy
SEASON All year
MAP Tom Harrison *Angeles Front Country*
PERMIT N/A

■ FEATURES

Whitney Canyon, tucked in the hills just off the busy freeway in Santa Clarita, appears dry and industrialized from the freeway off-ramp. But take an hour or two to explore the canyon and you'll discover a fine oak forest with a spring and seasonal waterfall.

■ DESCRIPTION

From the 14 Freeway east of Santa Clarita, take Exit 2 for eastbound Newhall Avenue. Immediately enter a large Park and Ride lot. Hiker parking can be found at the lower Whitney Canyon Park lot through a gate to the north (GPS N34° 21.878' W118° 30.044').

From the north end of the Whitney Canyon lot just before a bridge, go east on an unsigned dirt road leading into Whitney Canyon, which remains broad and uninteresting for the first half mile. Stay left as you pass two power-line service roads. You'll pass under some massive high-voltage power lines, and then the scenery improves. The canyon bottom narrows, and massive live oaks and sycamores arch overhead, creating inviting pools of shade, even on hot summer days. The gnarled appearance of the trees suggests that they are the survivors of multiple wildfires over decades and centuries.

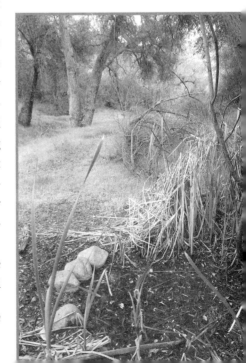

Pass a second set of large power lines. Just beyond an old wall

Artesian spring in Whitney Canyon

of light-colored masonry on the right, a small tributary canyon opens on the right (south) side, just shy of where the old road peters out, 1.0 mile from the start. Poke 30 yards into this little ravine, and you will soon come upon a cattail-choked freshwater marsh (GPS N34° 21.982' W118° 29.073'). A covey of quail might explode from this oasis as you approach it. In back of the marsh, look for an artesian sulfur spring—a clear pool of water, possibly with sulfurous bubbles coming up.

In the winter and spring, continue up the canyon on a narrower trail. Even if the lower canyon is dry, you'll likely start to see water flowing. Pass a series of cascades and eventually reach a lovely waterfall blocking farther progress up the canyon (1.7 miles; GPS N34° 22.183' W118° 28.552').

■ Hike 6 YERBA BUENA RIDGE ↗ 🐕 ☸

HIKE LENGTH 4.6 miles out-and-back; 1,400' elevation gain
DIFFICULTY Moderate
SEASON November–May
MAP Tom Harrison *Angeles Front Country*
PERMIT N/A

■ FEATURES

In the gentle hills above Little Tujunga Canyon are two delightful springs—little oak-sheltered recesses nestled in hills covered with chaparral. Both were largely spared by the 2009 Station Fire and the 2017 Creek Fire, although much of the surrounding slopes—particularly near the trailhead and around Yerba Buena Ridge—burned. Oak Spring lies in a shallow recess near the head of Oak Spring Canyon, just over the ridge from Gold Creek. Fascination Spring—one can only guess how it got this intriguing name—is hidden in a narrow crease on the south slope of the mountains, high above the Sunland-Tujunga Valley.

You start from Gold Creek, Little Tujunga's major tributary. As the name suggests, Gold Creek was once the scene of feverish mining activity. Most storied were the so-called Little Nugget placers, recovering gold right from the creekbed. The gold is gone, and this is ranch country now.

A good trail leads south from Gold Creek and climbs into the gentle hill country of Yerba Buena Ridge. A mile and a half up is Oak Spring, hidden in a small draw so that you don't see it until you're almost there. Then you climb up

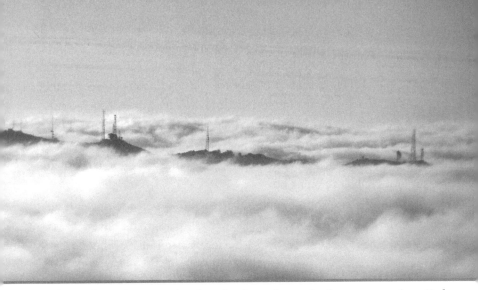

The Verdugo Mountains barely poke above the marine layer, as seen from Yerba Buena Ridge.

to Yerba Buena Ridge and optionally drop abruptly down to Fascination Spring. Oak Spring is shaded; the rest of the trip is through open chaparral. This is an ideal outing for a cool winter or spring day. Try it after a rain, when the springs bubble full and the aroma of damp chaparral perfumes the clean air.

■ DESCRIPTION

From the 210 Freeway in Lake View Terrace, take Exit 8 for Osborne Street. Turn right onto Foothill Boulevard and then left onto Osborne Street (after a mile Osborne Street becomes Little Tujunga Canyon Road). At 3.8 miles from the 210, turn right on Gold Creek Road. Continue 0.7 mile to signed Oak Spring Trail on the right (GPS N34° 19.130' W118° 20.015'), and park on the shoulder or at the Oak Springs Picnic Area just before the trail.

Proceed along the footpath across Gold Creek and up the chaparral-coated south slope that burned in the 2017 Creek Fire. Follow the trail as it makes one long switchback and then climbs south up the chaparral-covered hillside. Vistas open up over the wrinkled Gold Creek basin. The ranch you see down to the north was Paradise Ranch, scene of many a Cecil B. DeMille film extravaganza. Below to the east are the stone quarries where 770,000 tons of granite rock were removed for Hansen Dam from 1938 to 1940. In 1.25 miles you cross a divide and drop down to lush Oak Spring, where you'll find water except in the driest months. If it's a sunny day, the shade here is welcome. Remain on the trail as it crosses the creek and contours around the slope (south). This section of trail isn't as good as what you've just been over, but it's easily passable. Follow the trail through dense chaparral and burn area from the Station Fire, around the slope, across a small gully, and up to the Yerba Buena Ridge fire road (Forest Road 3N30; 2.3 miles). Here, you have a spectacular panorama southward over the Tujunga and San Fernando Valleys (GPS N34° 17.897' W118° 19.376'). Return the same way you came.

VARIATION It is possible to continue down to Fascination Spring, only interesting in the wet season. Walk 100 yards down the road—toward the city—and then take the signed Fascination Spring Trail dropping south (left) down the steep mountainside. The pathway here is narrow and at times hard to follow as it contours around the slope in a generally southwest direction, follows a ridge, and then reverses course eastward. At a junction marked by a post, stay left (east) and traverse into the next drainage. At the first switch-back near the ravine, it is possible to leave the trail and pick a path through the brush to Fascination Spring in the ravine (GPS N34° 17.544' W118° 19.391'). The spring was damaged by fire and erosion; now, most of the year, it is dry or nothing more than a damp patch above some riparian vegetation and is not worth the trouble to visit. The U.S. Forest Service hopes to eventually rehabilitate the spring. This variation adds 2.0 miles and 900 feet of elevation gain round-trip.

VARIATION You can make a wonderful loop with outstanding views of the Big Tujunga country by turning left up Yerba Buena Ridge Road (3N30). At the 3,892-foot-high point on the ridge, stay left to remain on the main road, and continue down to the wildly eroded Gold Canyon Saddle. Turn left again and descend Boulder Canyon Road to the unsigned Boulder Canyon Trail on the left. When it ends at Gold Creek Road, continue downhill past Repticular Ranch to your vehicle. This loop is 9 miles with 2,400 feet of elevation gain.

■ Hike 7 TRAIL CANYON FALLS ✈ ⊢ 🕴 🕴

HIKE LENGTH 4.5 miles out-and-back; 1,000' elevation gain
DIFFICULTY Moderate
SEASON December–May
MAP Tom Harrison *Angeles Front Country*
PERMIT N/A

Trail Canyon Falls

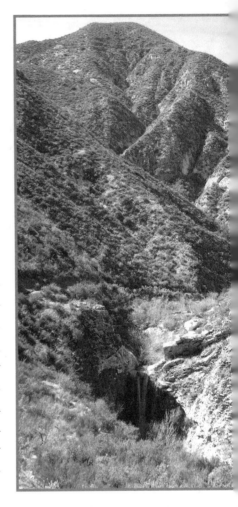

■ FEATURES

Trail Canyon cuts a deep swath through the western front country of the San Gabriels. Steep, chaparral-blanketed ridges surround it on both sides, and the great arched head of Condor Peak looms high on the eastern skyline. The scenic highlight is Trail Canyon Falls, 2 miles upcanyon, a delicate ribbon of whitewater swishing 30 feet into a cool sanctuary of alders and ferns. It used to be possible to continue upcanyon to Tom Lucas Trail Camp and on to Condor Peak, but the canyon above the falls burned in the 2009 Station Fire and is presently overgrown with a sea of ceanothus, leaving a nasty bushwhack and little trace of the old camp.

■ DESCRIPTION

From the 210 Freeway in Sunland, take Exit 11 for Sunland Boulevard. Go east 0.7 mile, as the road name changes to Foothill Boulevard; then turn left onto Oro Vista Avenue. Proceed 5.3 miles as the road becomes Big Tujunga Canyon Road. The trailhead is at mile marker 2.0. Park in the dirt turnout on the left (GPS N34° 18.226' W118° 15.490'), observing the sign that warns you not to block the gate on Forest Road 3N29. If the gate is open, you can drive 0.2 mile uphill to a fork, go right on FR 3N34, and continue 0.2 mile down to a parking area, saving 0.8 mile round-trip.

If the gate on FR 3N29 is closed at Big Tujunga Canyon Road, walk up the road to the aforementioned upper parking area. From this parking area, walk past the locked gate and follow the dirt road, passing some private cabins and crossing the creek. At 0.7 mile from Big Tujunga Canyon Road, stay right onto the signed Trail Canyon Trail. The trail briefly follows a tributary before dropping back into Trail Canyon and then following the bank, crossing the streambed several times. At 1.6 miles, climb onto the west wall to avoid a narrow, alder-choked section of the canyon. At 2.0 miles you round a sharp turn and then another turn, where the falls come into view, impressive as they plunge into the canyon depths below you. This is the best viewpoint along the trail. Just beyond where the trail again turns north, you will notice a narrow side path through the brush on which hikers could descend to a pool at the base of the falls—very steep and loose footing. Continuing on the main trail, you drop back into the canyon above the falls and reach the creek at the lip of the falls (GPS N34° 19.220' W118° 15.341'). This is a pleasant spot for a snack before retracing your steps.

VARIATION If you want to spend the night, continue 0.8 mile up to a small clearing above the creek, locally known as Lazy Tom Lucas Camp. The old Tom Lucas Trail Camp was more than a mile farther upcanyon, but it will be a struggle fighting through the brush unless the trail has been repaired.

■ Hike 8 MOUNT LUKENS VIA STONE CANYON TRAIL ↗ 🐕

HIKE LENGTH 8 miles out-and-back; 3,300' elevation gain

DIFFICULTY Strenuous

SEASON November–May

MAP Tom Harrison *Angeles Front Country*

PERMIT Post Adventure Pass or park outside fee area.

■ FEATURES

Mount Lukens (5,075'), a massive hogback mountain, lies just within the boundaries of Los Angeles, making it the highest point in the city. Years ago it was known as Sister Elsie Peak to commemorate the good deeds of a Roman Catholic nun in the Crescenta Valley. Sister Elsie, in charge of El Rancho de Dos Hermanas orphanage for Native American children, was much loved for her kind acts, particularly for nursing victims of a smallpox epidemic, during which she is reported to have lost her life. In the 1920s the U.S. Forest Service renamed the peak Mount Lukens in honor of Theodore P. Lukens, a onetime Angeles National Forest supervisor famed for his reforestation efforts at Henninger Flats. A fire lookout was built on the summit in 1923; in 1937 it was moved to nearby Josephine Peak because, even then, urban haze was interfering with observation.

This trip is the best and shortest way to climb Mount Lukens; it's the only way that is not via a long, monotonous fire road. But it is exceptionally steep. The old Stone Canyon Trail—not regularly maintained but readily passable—wastes no mileage in going from Big Tujunga to the summit; it proceeds right up the north slope, without a level stretch until you reach the summit ridge. Carry a bottle of water; you pass a sluggish spring about halfway up, but the water is not dependable.

■ **DESCRIPTION**

From the 210 Freeway in Sunland, take Exit 11 and go east on Sunland Boulevard. Go 0.7 mile as the road name changes to Foothill Boulevard, then turn left onto Oro Vista Avenue. Proceed 6.3 miles as the road becomes Big Tujunga Canyon Road. Near mile marker 3.0, turn right into the Wildwood Picnic Area and follow the road to its end at the Stone Canyon Trailhead (GPS N34° 17.621' W118° 14.331').

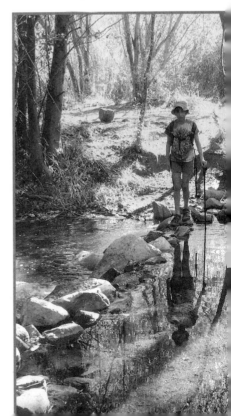

Follow the Stone Canyon Trail east 0.1 mile until you find a good place to ford Big Tujunga Creek (GPS N34° 17.588' W118° 14.248'). The crossing may be difficult if not impossible when the water is high. Finding the trail on the far side may be difficult as well—it parallels the south side of the creek and then switchbacks beneath a power-line pole and climbs the hillside onto a sloping bench left (east) of Stone Canyon Creek (GPS

Crossing Big Tujunga Creek during low flow. During high flow, the rocks are submerged.

N34° 17.545' W118° 14.189'). Once you locate the trail, there's no problem. Follow it as it zigzags steeply up the ridge left of Stone Canyon. At 2.0 miles you pass a small spring—a trickle of water during rainy season. At 3.8 miles you reach an old fire road on the ridge northwest of the summit. Turn left (southeast) and follow the bare path to the top (GPS N34° 16.125' W118° 14.302'). After enjoying the spectacular vista of the front-range country and the city (if the smog isn't too bad), return the way you came.

VARIATION You can make a wonderful 13-mile loop by descending the fire road on the east ridge, staying left at three junctions, to Grizzly Flats, then taking the Grizzly Flats Trail down to Stonyvale Picnic Area and walking back on Stonyvale Road to your vehicle.

■ Hike 9 CONDOR PEAK ⤢ 🐕

HIKE LENGTH 15 miles out-and-back; 3,400' elevation gain
DIFFICULTY Strenuous
SEASON November–May
MAP Tom Harrison *Angeles Front Country*
PERMIT N/A

■ FEATURES

There are no condors on Condor Peak, nor anywhere else in the San Gabriels today. The nearest redoubt of these magnificent birds is in the Sespe Creek area of Los Padres National Forest, some 50 miles northwest. Years ago, before humans disturbed its fragile habitat, this fast-vanishing species was common in all the Southern California mountains. According to mountain pioneer Faust Havermale, Condor Peak was so named because these monarchs of the air once nested here. Havermale wrote that he personally sighted 12 of these giant birds soaring around the peak in the early 20th century.

But nostalgia for the departed birds is not the only reason for climbing Condor Peak. From its airy summit, you get a breathtaking panorama over the rugged Big Tujunga country and beyond to the major peaks of the front range—Lukens to the south and Josephine, Strawberry, and San Gabriel to the southeast. The mile-high atmosphere is fresh, clean, and invigorating.

There is no shade on the entire route, so the trip should be done on a cool winter or spring day. Carry all the water you'll need; the one water source en route is not always flowing.

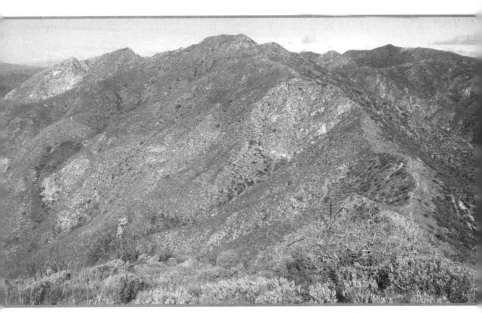

Condor Peak burned in the 2009 Station Fire, but chaparral is returning.

■ DESCRIPTION

From the 210 Freeway in Sunland, take Exit 11 and turn east on Sunland Boulevard. Go 0.7 mile, as the road name changes to Foothill Boulevard, then turn left onto Oro Vista Avenue. Proceed 7.8 miles as the road becomes Big Tujunga Canyon Road. Park in a dirt turnout on the right at mile marker 4.5 (0.1 mile beyond Vogel Flat; GPS N34° 17.259' W118° 13.487'), taking care not to block another gated fire road.

The unsigned and unlikely-looking trail begins on the north side of the road immediately opposite your parking turnout. It climbs steeply, then traverses 0.3 mile to join the Condor Peak Trail coming in from the east.

The trail zigzags up the divide between Vogel and Fusier Canyons; traverses a slope; and, at 2.3 miles, passes a small creek that usually has water in springtime. It continues up to the high ridge between the head of Vogel Canyon and Fox Creek, climbs steeply, and then contours around the west side of Fox Peak to Fox Saddle (5.8 miles). Continue northwest over false summits to a junction immediately east of the peak. A path on the right forks north toward Trail Canyon and Indian Ben Saddle, but our trail leads up the ridge to the true summit of Condor Peak (5,439'; GPS N34° 19.512' W118° 13.199'). Descend by the same route.

VARIATION It used to be possible to loop down Trail Canyon via Tom Lucas Camp, but the upper canyon was ravaged in the 2009 Station Fire and is currently a horrible bushwhack. If the U.S. Forest Service indicates the trail has been cleared, it is a worthy 16-mile trip with a 2.5-mile car or bicycle shuttle between trailheads.

Fox Peak (5,033') is an easy climb from the saddle to the northwest, with 350 feet of elevation gain over 0.2 mile on a use trail.

■ Hike 10 MOUNT LUKENS VIA HAINES CANYON TRAIL ↗ 🐐 ☸

HIKE LENGTH 10 miles out-and-back; 2,800' elevation gain
DIFFICULTY Strenuous
SEASON November–May
MAP Tom Harrison *Angeles Front Country*
PERMIT N/A

■ FEATURES

Mount Lukens is laced with enjoyable trails and fire roads that offer a vigorous workout and fantastic views. This trip approaches the mountain from the south. In former editions of this book, it used the Sister Elsie Trail, which nearly vanished after the Station Fire. Now you are better off taking the Old

On the Blue Bug Trail

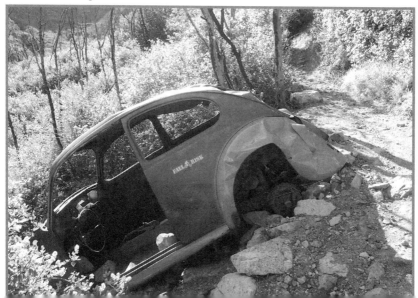

Mount Lukens Trail, which is beloved and well maintained by mountain bikers. There is little shade en route, so do it on a cool winter or spring day.

■ DESCRIPTION

From the 210 Freeway in Tujunga, take Exit 16 to head north on Lowell Avenue. In 0.6 mile, turn left (northwest) on Foothill Boulevard. In 0.9 mile, turn right on Haines Canyon Avenue. Proceed 0.9 mile to the end (GPS N34° 15.652' W118° 16.692'), briefly jogging right along the way. Backtrack to find a place to park on the shoulder, observing parking restrictions.

Walk up the road beyond the gate. Stay on the main road, passing a paved private road on the left and a debris basin. The trail soon deteriorates to a singletrack. At 1.2 miles, the abandoned Haines Canyon Motorway curves right and climbs out of the canyon. You could take this route, but it's more fun to stay left in the canyon on trail that follows the east side of the creek.

At 1.9 miles, reach a spring feeding the creek (beware of poison oak). The unsigned old Sister Elsie Trail crosses the creek here and climbs to join the Stone Canyon Trail on the shoulder of Mount Lukens (see Hike 8). It is currently in poor condition, so unless you are a glutton for punishment, you'll prefer staying right on the Old Mount Lukens Trail (also known as the Blue Bug Trail in honor of a striking car wreck near the top).

At 2.9 miles, join the upper part of the Haines Canyon Motorway (Forest Road 2N76). Follow it up to meet the Stone Canyon Trail on the west shoulder of Mount Lukens (4.5 miles; 4,930'), where views open northward across the mighty gorge of Big Tujunga. Turn right and finish the short final stretch to the antenna-studded summit (GPS N34° 16.125' W118° 14.302'). Return the way you came, or use the Haines Canyon Motorway to loop back.

VARIATION To make a great 9.5-mile loop hike, follow the Mount Lukens Truck Trail down the east ridge of Lukens 1.1 miles, then turn right onto the Pickens Spur road (FR 2N76C) that narrows to become the Crescenta View Trail and switchbacks down to the Deukmejian Wilderness Park. Turn left onto the Dunsmore Creek Trail, an old fire road, and follow it to the trailhead on Markridge Road. You'll need a 2.7-mile car, bicycle, or ride-sharing shuttle to get back to Haines Canyon.

■ Hike 11 LOWER ARROYO SECO ↗ 🐕 👫 ⊛ 🥾

HIKE LENGTH 5 miles out-and-back; 300' elevation gain

DIFFICULTY Easy

SEASON November–May

MAP Tom Harrison *Angeles Front Country*

PERMIT N/A

■ FEATURES

Today the Arroyo Seco is largely bypassed and forgotten, but in the Great Hiking Era it was one of the most popular vacation spots in the range. Under its luxuriant cover of willows, sycamores, alders, and bays, the canyon reverberated with the lusty shouts and merry songs of hikers and campers. The lower reaches were dotted with rustic cabins and well-used picnic spots. This was before the Angeles Crest Highway provided ready access into the mountains, climbing high on the west slope of the canyon. Now nature's stillness reigns supreme in the canyon, broken only by the gentle murmur of the stream, the soft rustle of sycamore leaves, and—as a reminder of civilization's nearness—the occasional muffled roar of an automobile rounding a curve far above.

In 1911, J. R. Phillips fashioned a tourist resort, old Camp Oak Wilde, about halfway up this great gorge on a forested streamside bench. For almost three decades, until it was nearly obliterated in the 1938 flood, this was a favorite spot of vacationing Southlanders. In the 1920s a road was built up the lower Arroyo Seco to the camp; it too was severely damaged in the

Lower Arroyo Seco is shaded by gnarled oaks.

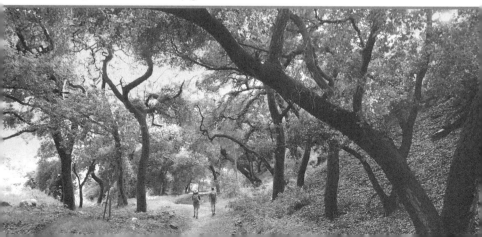

greatest torrent ever known in the San Gabriels. The 2009 Station Fire ravaged the area yet again. Today only remnants of the road remain, and a few stone foundations at Oakwilde are the only signs of what once went on here. Time and nature's gradual healing process have restored much of the beauty of the Arroyo Seco. Although parts of the lower canyon have been permanently marred by man's work—most notably the Brown Canyon Debris Dam—there is much to be seen and enjoyed in this great canyon. This trail trip gives you a fair sampling.

■ DESCRIPTION

From the 210 Freeway in Pasadena, take Exit 22B to go north on Windsor Avenue. In 0.8 mile, park at a busy lot on the left where Windsor meets Ventura Street (GPS N34° 11.665' W118° 10.077').

You will notice two paved roads—both with gates usually locked—leading north down toward the canyon entrance. Take the right (eastern) of the two; the left road goes to the Jet Propulsion Laboratory parking lot. Proceed on foot down the road, which gains the Arroyo Seco entrance in 0.6 mile. You pass the assorted markings of the Pasadena Water Department—fences, retaining walls, gauging stations, and a host of warning signs—and reach U.S. Forest Service residences in 1.2 miles. Go left at a road fork; now the canyon closes in and the scenery becomes more woodsy—giant canyon oaks, alders, willows, sycamores, and even a few eucalyptus trees from resort days. This route is for both hikers and equestrians, so you'll most likely pass horseback riders. The trail alternates between following the old road and stream-hopping where the roadbed and bridges have washed out.

As the canyon narrows, you pass Teddy's Outpost Picnic Area, named for a small roadside resort operated by Theodore "Teddy" Syvertson from 1914 to 1926. At 2.5 miles you reach the Gould Mesa Campground, honoring Will Gould, who homesteaded here in the 1890s, and just beyond, a side road leading up to Gould Mesa and the Angeles Crest Highway (GPS N34° 13.342' W118° 10.704'). This is a good turnaround point.

VARIATION If you have time, there's plenty more to see up the canyon. Nino Picnic Area is 0.4 mile farther. Above Nino the canyon narrows, twists, and turns, and remnants of the old road become less evident. In another 1.1 miles you reach Paul Little Memorial Picnic Area on the left. Going right, the trail climbs up the steep east slope of the canyon to get around Brown Canyon

Debris Dam, and then drops back into the gorge and rounds two sharp bends before reaching Oakwilde, 5.4 miles from the start. Little remains of the old road's-end resort or the Oakwilde Trail Camp that replaced it. The Dark Canyon Trail once led up to the Angeles Crest Highway from here, but it was obliterated by landslide and fire. The Ken Burton Trail, popular with sturdy mountain bikers, climbs to the Brown Mountain Fire Road, which you could follow back to El Prieto Canyon for an excellent 15-mile loop.

■ Hike 12 DOWN THE ARROYO SECO ↗ 🐕 ◉ 🚶

HIKE LENGTH 10 miles one-way; 700' elevation gain, 2,700' elevation loss
DIFFICULTY Moderate
SEASON November–May
MAP Tom Harrison *Angeles Front Country*
PERMIT Post Adventure Pass at Switzer, or park outside fee area.

■ FEATURES

This trip makes the outstanding descent of the Arroyo Seco from Switzer Picnic Area to Pasadena along the western part of the Gabrielino Trail. En

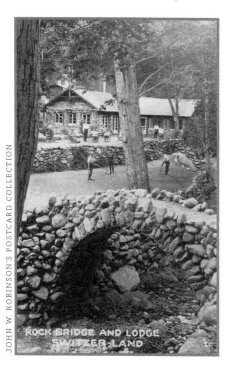

route, it passes through the sites of three once-famous mountain resorts: Switzer's Camp, Camp Oak Wilde, and Teddy's Outpost. To avoid the difficult middle gorge of the Arroyo Seco, known as Royal Gorge, the trail climbs up and over chaparral-blanketed ridges, which are not very pleasant to walk on a hot day; do it when the weather is cool. The Arroyo Seco burned so badly in the 2009 Station Fire that it did not fully reopen until 2018. However, the riparian vegetation has recovered quickly, as it has after many fires and floods before.

Switzer Camp (circa 1928)

JOHN W. ROBINSON'S POSTCARD COLLECTION

■ DESCRIPTION

This trip requires a 15-mile car shuttle or ride-sharing trip. Leave your get-away vehicle at the south end. From the 210 Freeway in Pasadena, take Exit 22B north on Windsor Avenue. In 0.8 mile, park at a busy lot on the left where Windsor meets Ventura Street (GPS N34° 11.665' W118° 10.077'). To reach the north end, return to the 210 and go right (west) to CA 2 (Exit 20). Drive 10 miles north up CA 2 to the turnoff for Switzer Picnic Area on the right (mile marker 2 LA 34.2). Continue down the paved access road 0.5 mile to the parking lot next to the picnic area (GPS N34° 15.969' W118° 08.718'). (If the lot is full or the access road happens to be closed and gated, you can park at the top and walk down into the picnic area—250 feet of elevation loss in 0.5 mile.)

From the west end of the Switzer Picnic Area, start hiking on the Gabrielino Trail at a sign for Switzer Falls. Make your way across the bridge and along a road past outlying picnic tables, and then down along the alder-shaded stream. Soon nothing but the clear-flowing stream and rustling leaves disturb the silence. Remnants of an old paved road are occasionally underfoot. In a couple of spots, you ford the stream by boulder-hopping—no problem except after heavy rain.

One mile down the canyon, you come upon the foundation remnants of Switzer's Camp, now a remote picnic area. The main trail crosses to the west side of the creek at Switzer's Camp. Don't be lured onto one of the use trails continuing down the east side to crumbling cliffs above Switzer Falls, where many fatal accidents have occurred. Watch for the foundations of Christ Chapel on the cliff high above the falls.

Walk down to a fork in the trail at 1.3 miles. You will probably hear, if not clearly see, the 50-foot cascade known as Switzer Falls to the east. It is worth the short detour if the water is running well. Our way continues on the right fork (Gabrielino Trail), which now begins a mile-long traverse through chaparral. This less than perfectly scenic stretch avoids a narrow, twisting trench called Royal Gorge, through which the Arroyo Seco stream tumbles and sometimes abruptly drops.

At 2.6 miles, the trail joins a shady tributary of Long Canyon, and later joins Long Canyon itself, replete with a trickling stream. The trail mostly clings to a narrow ledge cut at great effort into the east wall of the canyon. Alongside the trail you'll discover at least five kinds of ferns, plus mosses, miner's lettuce, poison oak, and Humboldt lilies (in bloom during early summer).

At 3.9 miles, the waters of Long Canyon swish down through a sculpted grotto to join Arroyo Seco. The trail descends to Arroyo Seco canyon's narrow floor and stays there, crossing and recrossing many times over the next few miles. At 5.2 miles, pass the signed Ken Burton Trail on the left, favored by mountain bikers. The trail may disappear in the wash, but just continue downstream through the gorgeous gorge flanked by soaring walls and dappled with shade cast by the ever-present alders. Big-leaf maples put on a great show here in November, their bright yellow leaves boldly contrasting with the earthy greens, grays, and browns of the canyon's dimly lit bottom. Camp Oak Wilde, operated by J. R. Phillips, stood here from 1911 until it was destroyed by flood in 1938. The Oakwilde Campground was rebuilt in the same place but was wiped out by the Station Fire. You can still find flat ground to camp here if you wish; treat the streamwater before drinking.

The canyon widens a bit. At 5.9 miles, your way is abruptly blocked by the large Brown Canyon Debris Dam. Built in the 1940s to reduce the flow of detritus into Pasadena, it has filled up and no longer serves its purpose but remains as a scar on the canyon that will take nature many more years to demolish. Just short of the dam, the trail climbs onto the east wall of the canyon, bypasses the dam, and descends steeply to reach the canyon bottom at a sign for the Paul Little Memorial Picnic Area.

The hardest work is over, and a decent path takes you down the remainder of the gently sloping canyon. Pass the Nino Picnic Area. The trail gradually improves into a road and crosses several bridges in varying states of repair. At 8.1 miles, pass the busy Gould Mesa Campground, named for Will Gould, a homesteader who lived here in the 1890s. After Teddy's Outpost Picnic Area and the south end of the burn area, watch for a gauging station on the right and some U.S. Forest Service residences on the left. The last segment of the trail is paved and you are likely to run into cyclists, joggers, parents pushing strollers, and even skateboarders. Pass the imposing complex of Caltech's Jet Propulsion Laboratory on the right, and eventually emerge at the Arroyo Boulevard trailhead.

■ Hike 13 SWITZER FALLS 🥾 🐕 👫 ⊛

HIKE LENGTH 3.6 miles out-and-back; 700' elevation gain

DIFFICULTY Easy

SEASON November–June

MAP Tom Harrison *Angeles Front Country*

PERMIT Post Adventure Pass, or park outside fee area.

■ FEATURES

Once, the name Switzer was almost synonymous with Arroyo Seco. This was when Switzer Camp was the most famous trail resort in the range. By foot, by horse, or by burro, hundreds of people traveled up the Arroyo Seco every weekend to visit this picturesque, woodsy hostelry above Switzer Falls.

It was Commodore Perry Switzer—along with the mountain-loving Watermans, Bob and Liz—who fashioned this wilderness resort back in 1884. Twice weekly, Switzer led his burro train up the tortuous Arroyo Seco Trail, with its 60 stream crossings and endless switchbacks. A cow horn was left dangling on a manzanita bush half a mile below camp, with printed instructions to issue forth a blast for each hungry guest. When the tired visitors finally reached camp, they would find a sizzling dinner awaiting them. Trout from the adjacent stream were featured.

It was under hospitable Lloyd and Bertha Austin (1912–1936) that Switzer's really became the number one resort in the range. The warmth and friendliness of the Austins attracted thousands from

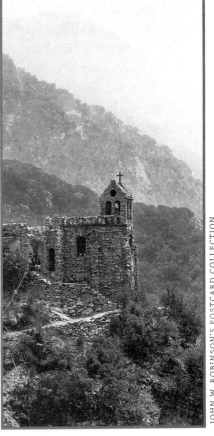

JOHN W. ROBINSON'S POSTCARD COLLECTION

Switzer's Chapel (1924–1959)

all walks of life. Among those who signed the guest register were Henry Ford, Shirley Temple, Clark Gable, and Mary Pickford. LEAVE YOUR CARES AND ANIMALS THIS SIDE OF THE STREAM was the sign that greeted approaching visitors; another sign over the lodge door read THE AUSTIN HOME . . . AND YOURS. So that his guests would have the opportunity for a variety of experiences, Lloyd added tennis and croquet courts, a well-stocked library, a playground, an open-air dance floor for Switzer Saturday Nights, and a miniature Christ Chapel perched above the falls for Sunday morning worship.

All this is gone now, the victim of progress in the form of the Angeles Crest Highway. With people able to drive in minutes to places that once required hours or days of strenuous hiking, the old camp lost its wilderness appeal. After withering for two decades, it was finally abandoned and all buildings removed in 1959. The sylvan bench just above the falls became Commodore Switzer Trail Camp and now has become simply a picnic area with no overnight camping.

This trip is a delightful streamside stroll under alder, oak, maple, and sycamore trees. You visit the old campsite and then descend into the narrow Royal Gorge of the Arroyo Seco for a close-up view of plunging Switzer Falls and the numerous little pools and cascades that dot the shady chasm. (Don't try to climb the falls; many have been injured in the attempt.)

■ DESCRIPTION

Exit the 210 Freeway at Angeles Crest Highway (Highway 2) in La Cañada Flintridge. Drive 10 miles north to the turnoff for Switzer Picnic Area on the right (mile marker 2 LA 34.2). Drive 0.5 mile down the paved access road to the parking lot next to the picnic area, where the road makes a hairpin turn (GPS N34° 15.969' W118° 08.718'). (If the access road is closed and gated, park at the top and walk to the picnic area—250 feet of elevation loss in 0.5 mile.)

Cross the bridge and follow the trail downcanyon 1.0 mile to Commodore Switzer Trail Camp. Rock-hop across the stream, and follow the trail as it climbs and then contours along the west slope above the falls. Do *not* follow the creek below camp; it abruptly drops 50 feet at the falls. Reach a trail junction at 1.3 miles: the right (southwest) fork is the main Gabrielino Trail down to Oakwilde and Pasadena (see Hike 12). Go left (southeast) on the Bear Canyon Trail, dropping into the gorge of the Arroyo Seco below the falls. When you reach the creek, turn left and walk upstream to Switzer

Falls (1.8 miles). Remember, don't climb the sheer rock sidewalls of the falls. Return the way you came.

■ Hike 14 DAWN MINE ⟳ 🐕 🏃

HIKE LENGTH 6-mile loop; 1,500' elevation gain

DIFFICULTY Moderate

SEASON November–May

MAP Tom Harrison *Angeles Front Country*

PERMIT N/A

■ FEATURES

Woodsy Millard Canyon ranks as one of the more pleasant retreats in the front range of the San Gabriels. Nestled between Sunset Ridge and Brown Mountain, the canyon seldom suffers the full glare of sunlight. Beneath overarching oaks and sycamores, the small stream glides and dances over water-tempered boulders, finally to tumble over Millard Canyon Falls.

Deep in the upper reaches of Millard Canyon are the remains of Dawn Mine, the most storied gold prospect in the front range. Gold was discovered here in 1895, and the ore-bearing veins were worked on and off with varying degrees of success into the early 1950s. No great amount of gold was ever recovered, despite repeated boasts of imminent bonanzas by overly optimistic prospectors.

Since the Station Fire, volunteer trail crews have reopened the trail up Millard Canyon to Dawn Mine. The canyon is a sylvan delight, where you can temporarily forget your proximity to civilization. It is a peaceful place to while away the hours, to saunter rather than stride.

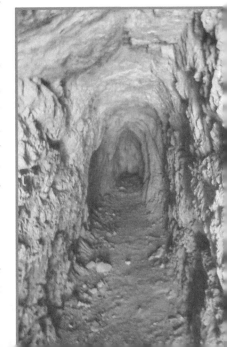

Exploratory adit at Dawn Mine, photographed from the mouth. Beware of entering old mine shafts, which have been known to collapse.

■ DESCRIPTION

From the 210 Freeway in Pasadena, take Exit 23 for Lincoln Avenue. Go north on Lincoln for 1.8 miles, then turn right on Loma Alta Drive. Proceed 0.6 mile east to Chaney Trail (a paved road) on the left. Drive past a sturdy gate, typically open 6 a.m.–8 p.m., and proceed sharply uphill 1.1 miles to the road crest at Sunset Ridge, where there's parking space by the roadside (GPS N34° 12.884' W118° 08.851'). If you are here on the weekend and this small parking area is full, your best bet is to continue another 0.5 mile down to the bottom of Millard Canyon.

Hike up the Sunset Ridge fire road, where you will almost immediately see a branch of the Sunset Ridge Trail on the left coming up from the Millard Canyon parking area. Stay on the paved fire road to another intersection with the marked Sunset Ridge Trail leading left at 0.3 mile. Follow this trail around the ridge and down into Millard Canyon above the falls. Just before you reach the canyon bottom, at a trail junction at 0.8 mile, go left (the right branch leads back up to Sunset Ridge fire road). When the trail reaches the streambed near a historic cabin, it all but disappears in a jumble of boulders.

If time permits, take a 0.1-mile detour downstream to the top of Millard Canyon Falls. Then follow whatever trail you can upstream, staying in the main canyon, to the woodsy haunt that once was Dawn Mine (2.2 miles; GPS N34° 13.565' W118° 07.778'). Not much remains—scattered diggings, pieces of rusted mill machinery, and a narrow tunnel entrance. Do not try to explore the tunnel; there are difficult-to-detect water-filled holes. On the southeast side of the canyon, look for the foundation and metal stilts that supported prospector Michael Ryan's house on an airy promontory above the creek. A second, taller adit can be found on the north wall of the canyon by boulder-hopping up the creek 0.1 mile.

To close the loop, look for a trail opposite the mine climbing the southeast wall of the canyon. Ryan originally built this trail for his mules Jack and Jill to haul ore out of the canyon to the railway. It has been heavily reworked by the volunteer Restoration Legacy Crew, but it still involves a narrow cliff-hanging segment that might be uncomfortable for some hikers. When you reach the Mount Lowe Railway bed at Dawn Station (2.8 miles), turn right and head down Sunset Ridge. The most direct route stays on the wide road, while the harder but more scenic Sunset Ridge Trail forks to the right below a rocky knob known as the Cape of Good Hope and hangs on the canyon wall between the road and the canyon bottom before reaching the historic cabin you originally passed and climbing back to Sunset Ridge.

■ Hike 15 MILLARD CANYON FALLS

HIKE LENGTH 1.2 miles out-and-back; 250' elevation gain
DIFFICULTY Easy
SEASON November–May
MAP Tom Harrison *Angeles Front Country*
PERMIT Post Adventure Pass.

■ FEATURES

Millard Canyon's 50-foot falls are wedged snugly where the lower canyon narrows, about 0.5 mile above the Millard Canyon picnic area. The short

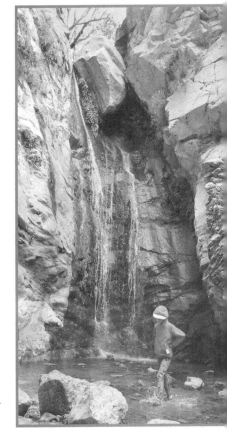

canyon-bottom walk is shaded most of the way by huge canyon oaks and a handful of tall alders and willows. The many stream crossings and boulders form a natural jungle gym for little hikers. Only a short distance from Altadena, this route makes an ideal Sunday-afternoon saunter.

■ DESCRIPTION

From the 210 Freeway, take Exit 23 for Lincoln Avenue. Drive north on Lincoln 1.8 miles, and turn right on Loma Alta Drive. Go 0.6 mile east to Chaney Trail (a paved road) on the left. Drive 1.7 miles to the road's end at a large parking lot along Millard Creek (GPS N34° 12.982' W118° 08.733'),

Even the winter chill isn't enough to keep a young hiker from splashing beneath Millard Canyon Falls.

passing a sturdy gate that is typically open from 6 a.m. to 8 p.m. and crossing Sunset Ridge.

Pass a locked gate and proceed a hundred yards up the fire road to Millard Canyon Trail Camp. At the upper end of the campground, a wooden sign points right (east) to Millard Canyon Falls. Follow the shady canyon trail 0.6 mile to the foot of the falls (GPS N34° 13.137' W118° 08.513'). Don't try to climb over the falls; people have been injured here.

Return the way you came.

■ Hike 16 BROWN MOUNTAIN LOOP ⟳ 🐐

HIKE LENGTH 12-mile loop; 3,000' elevation gain

DIFFICULTY Strenuous

SEASON November–May

MAP Tom Harrison *Angeles Front Country*

PERMIT N/A

■ FEATURES

The Brown Boys—Owen and Jason—were familiar figures in and around the foothills of the front range back in the 1880s. These long-bearded sons of fiery pre–Civil War abolitionist John Brown lived in a small log cabin near the head of El Prieto Canyon, a beautiful wooded glen between the Arroyo Seco and Millard Canyon. Great lovers of nature, the men spent much time exploring the neighboring mountains. They sought out a mountain peak to name in honor of their famous father. After an unsuccessful attempt to place his name on

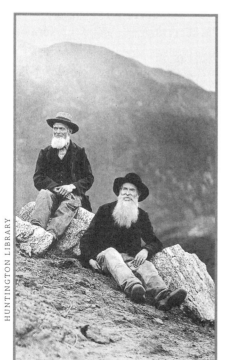

Owen and Jason Brown, two sons of John Brown, on Brown Mountain (circa 1884)

HUNTINGTON LIBRARY

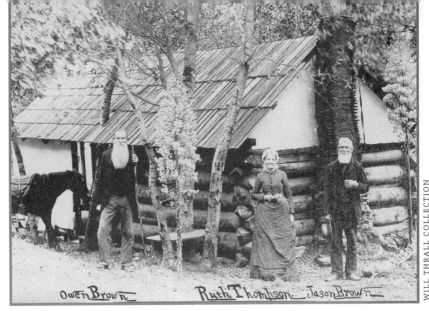

The Brown Boys at their El Prieto Cabin (circa 1887)

what later became known as Mount Lowe, they settled on the long, rounded mountain rising high between Millard Canyon and Bear Creek. Today it is still known as Brown Mountain.

This lengthy loop trip climbs up Millard Canyon to Tom Sloan Saddle (named for a former district ranger), traverses the 4,485-foot hogback of Brown Mountain, and descends from the west ridge around the south slope back to the starting point. You should be in good physical condition for this one, and because part of the loop is trailless, wear lug-soled boots. The area burned in the 2009 Station Fire, but the trail from Millard to Tom Sloan was rebuilt by the volunteer Restoration Legacy Crew.

■ DESCRIPTION

From the 210 Freeway, take Exit 23 for Lincoln Avenue. Go north on Lincoln Avenue for 1.8 miles, then turn right on Loma Alta Drive. Proceed 0.6 mile east to Chaney Trail (a paved road) on the left. Drive past a sturdy gate that is typically open from 6 a.m. to 8 p.m., and proceed 1.1 miles sharply uphill to the road crest at Sunset Ridge, where there's roadside parking (GPS N34° 12.884' W118° 08.851'). If you are here on the weekend and this small parking area is full, your best bet is to continue another 0.5 mile down to the bottom of Millard Canyon.

Hike up the Sunset Ridge fire road about 400 yards (passing a branch of the Sunset Ridge Trail down to Millard Campground) to the signed Sunset

Ridge Trail leading left, around the ridge into Millard Canyon above the falls (see Hike 14). Follow the streamside trail, hopping boulders where the footpath has been washed out, to the Dawn Mine (2.1 miles). Continue upstream to where the creek splits (2.5 miles); look for the easily missed trail on the right side of the left fork, and switchback up it to Tom Sloan Saddle, 3.6 miles from the start. Here, you stand on the divide between Millard Canyon and Bear Creek, at a five-way trail junction (see Hike 29). From the saddle, scramble left (west) up the firebreak and a faint hikers' footpath, climbing over or around three false summits, to the true hogback summit of Brown Mountain (4.7 miles; GPS N34° 14.208' W118° 08.831'). The small burn along the ridge was caused by a 2017 lightning strike.

Standing on the bare summit, you are rewarded with a superb panorama of the front range. To the west, across the yawning chasm of the Arroyo Seco, is Mount Lukens. Northward, beyond Bear Creek and the upper Arroyo Seco, are the impressive humps of Josephine and Strawberry Peaks. Eastward are the triumvirate of San Gabriel Peak, Mount Markham, and Mount Lowe. And to the south, past Millard Canyon, sprawls the megalopolis, sometimes half hidden in brown murkiness.

When you're through savoring the view, continue west along the firebreak, dropping 1,600 feet to the upper end of the Brown Mountain fire road (closed to public vehicles) and the top of the Ken Burton Trail (6.2 miles). Turn left and proceed down the fire road as it curves southeastward around the lower slopes of Brown Mountain. Go left (east) at all road junctions. The fire road reaches the Millard Canyon Trail Camp at 11.0 miles. Because your car is up on Sunset Ridge, you'll have to take the Sunset Ridge Trail from the lower end of the campground 400 feet up the other side of the canyon back to your vehicle (11.8 miles).

■ Hike 17 MOUNT LOWE TRAIL CAMP FROM SUNSET RIDGE ◉ ⊶ ⊛ 🚶

HIKE LENGTH 11-mile loop; 2,600' elevation gain
DIFFICULTY Strenuous (1 day); moderate (2 days)
SEASON November–May
MAP Tom Harrison *Angeles Front Country*
PERMIT N/A

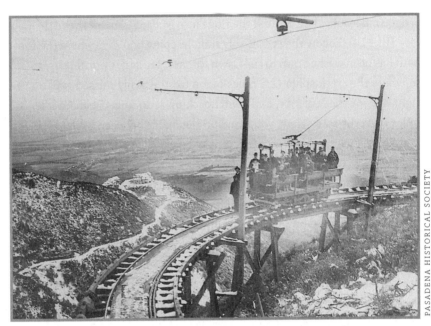

The Grand Circular Bridge on the Mount Lowe Railway (1895)

PASADENA HISTORICAL SOCIETY

■ FEATURES

The Mount Lowe Scenic Railway was one of the early 20th century's engineering marvels, visited by an estimated 3 million people during its 43 years of operation (1893–1936). This trip climbs the Sunset Ridge Trail, above Millard Canyon, to the old railway bed near what was once called the Cape of Good Hope. The route then follows the railway bed, now the Sunset Ridge–Mount Lowe fire road, to the Mount Lowe Tavern site, now the Mount Lowe Trail Camp. The old railway bed is gently graded and offers a splendid panorama over mountain, canyon, and lowland—particularly on a clear winter or spring day when air pollution does not muddy the sky. You will pass some of the "stations" denoting historic sites on the old railroad, with signs and plaques erected by weekend volunteers of the Scenic Mount Lowe Railway Historical Committee. The loop portion of this hike overlaps with the loop of Hike 18, and both are excellent outings.

You can make this a strenuous one-day trip or stay overnight at Mount Lowe Trail Camp, making it a pleasant two-day outing. *Note:* The water at Mount Lowe Trail Camp may dry up in the summer and should be filtered or boiled before use.

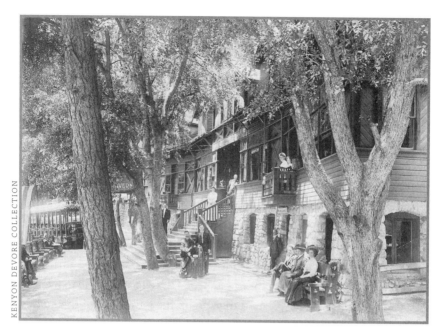

Ye Alpine Tavern, Mount Lowe Railway (circa 1914)

■ **DESCRIPTION**

From the 210 Freeway, take Exit 23 for Lincoln Avenue. Go north on Lincoln Avenue for 1.8 miles, then turn right on Loma Alta Drive. Proceed 0.6 mile east to Chaney Trail (a paved road) on the left. Drive past a sturdy gate that is typically open from 6 a.m. to 8 p.m., and proceed 1.1 miles sharply uphill to the road crest at Sunset Ridge, where there's roadside parking (GPS N34° 12.884' W118° 08.851'). If you are here on the weekend and this small parking area is full, your best bet is to continue another 0.5 mile down to the bottom of Millard Canyon.

Walk past the locked gate and up the fire road 0.3 mile (passing a branch of the Sunset Ridge Trail down to Millard Campground) to a junction on your left. Take the signed Sunset Ridge Trail, which contours around the ridge above Millard Canyon. Just before you reach the canyon bottom is a trail junction (0.8 mile). Go right (the left branch goes to the floor of Millard Canyon) and follow the trail all the way up to the top of Sunset Ridge (2.7 miles), where you rejoin the fire road. As you proceed up the fire road, Echo Mountain and its historical ruins come into view down to your right. Meet the old railway bed coming up from Echo Mountain. Just beyond, you pass a metal post (the first of the "stations") on your left, indicating that you have reached Cape of Good Hope, where the mountain railroad rounded a point above Millard Canyon.

At 3.0 miles you pass the Dawn Mine Trail, leading left down into Millard Canyon (an option on your return; see Hike 14), and then to Dawn Mine Station, Grand Circular Bridge (3.5 miles), and Horseshoe Curve (4.0 miles) as the route climbs high along the east wall of Millard Canyon. Finally, the old roadbed turns east, passes through Granite Gate (4.4 miles), ascends to near the head of Grand Canyon, and reaches Mount Lowe Trail Camp on your left, 5.3 miles from the start (GPS N34° 13.588' W118° 06.592'). The shady trail camp—on the site of old Mount Lowe Tavern—is equipped with tables, stoves, restrooms, and a spring-fed cistern (treat water.

To make a partial loop, continue up the roadway and then turn right at a junction to Inspiration Point (5.7 miles). Descend via Castle Canyon to Echo Mountain (see Hike 18), and then go up the lower part of the railway bed to Sunset Ridge (8.3 miles). Return the way you came or simply follow the Sunset Ridge fire road all the way down.

VARIATION Another loop option is to take the unmarked Tom Sloan Trail, rebuilt in 2018, from Mount Lowe Trail Camp to Tom Sloan Saddle, and then follow another restored trail down to Dawn Mine and out via Millard Canyon or Sunset Ridge (see Hike 14). This variation is also 11 miles.

■ Hike 18 MOUNT LOWE RAILWAY LOOP TOUR ○ 🐕 ⊛ 🚶

HIKE LENGTH 11-mile loop; 2,800' elevation gain
DIFFICULTY Strenuous (1 day); moderate (2 days)
SEASON November–May
MAP Tom Harrison *Angeles Front Country*
PERMIT N/A

■ FEATURES

In the early decades of the 20th century, the Mount Lowe Railway attracted tourists by the thousands. No visit to Southern California was complete without taking the thrilling ride up the cable incline to Echo Mountain, and then the twisting trolley trip to rustic Ye Alpine Tavern, nestled deep in a forest cove on the slopes of Mount Lowe. When the mountain railway was built, it was considered one of the engineering wonders of the world.

The Mount Lowe Railway and resort complex was the idea of two visionary Pasadenans: Civil War balloonist and inventor Thaddeus S. C. Lowe and engineer David J. Macpherson. With Lowe supplying the capital and Macpherson directing operations, the railway was hacked out of the mountainside in three stages from 1892 to 1895. First was a trolley line from Altadena into Rubio Canyon, where the first of Lowe's popular edifices, Rubio Pavilion, was located (see Hike 20). Then an incline railway climbed 1,300 feet to Echo Mountain, where two hostelries—The Chalet and Echo Mountain House—were perched (see Hike 19). Finally, a 4-mile winding trolley ride, past airy viewpoints such as Horseshoe Curve, Cape of Good Hope, Grand Circular Bridge, and Granite Gate, carried awestruck visitors to Ye Alpine Tavern (later called Mount Lowe Tavern). Lowe was bankrupted by the venture, and for most of the 43 years of its operation, the Pacific Electric Railway Company ran the complex. From its opening in 1893 until the burning of Mount Lowe Tavern in 1936, the renowned mountain railway and resort complex was visited by an estimated 3 million people.

Above Echo Mountain, the scars of the winding railway are clearly visible, and it is possible to hike to the tavern site along its broken bed, the

The Granite Gate on the Mount Lowe Railway (circa 1915)

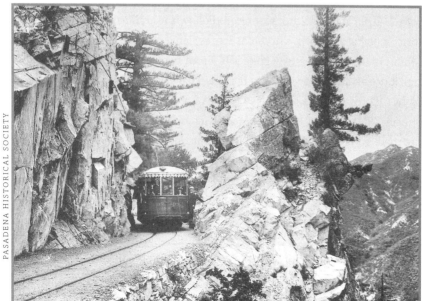

upper section of which is now part of the Sunset Ridge–Mount Lowe fire road (see Hike 17). At the old tavern site, under spreading oaks and big-cone Douglas-firs, the U.S. Forest Service has constructed the Mount Lowe Trail Camp, with tables, stoves, restrooms, and a spring-fed cistern (treat water).

A half mile south of the trail camp, overlooking the San Gabriel Valley, is the ramada at Inspiration Point, where tourists took in the view that was described in Mount Lowe Railway days as breathtaking, beautiful, and inspiring.

Over the years, much restoration work has been accomplished by weekend volunteers of the Scenic Mount Lowe Railway Historical Committee. Old trails have been cleared, artifacts have been uncovered and placed on display at Echo Mountain, and—their crowning achievement—the ramada at Inspiration Point was rebuilt and dedicated in 1996.

Hikers with vivid imaginations can stand among the foundations of the mountain railway and picture themselves a part of Professor Lowe's dream come true. This loop trip is for those with such imaginations.

■ DESCRIPTION

From the 210 Freeway in Pasadena, take Exit 26 for Lake Avenue. Go north on Lake Avenue for 3.6 miles to where the street bends left and becomes Loma Alta Drive (GPS N34° 12.236' W118° 07.832'). Look for curbside parking near this intersection.

To your right (east), near a large locked gate, is the beginning of the Sam Merrill Trail to Echo Mountain. Follow the trail east through the historic Cobb Estate, down across Las Flores Canyon, and up the slopes to Echo Mountain at 2.7 miles (see Hike 19). From Echo Mountain, backtrack to a trail junction and follow the broad, graded railway bed north around the head of Las Flores Canyon to Sunset Ridge (3.5 miles), where you pick up the Sunset Ridge–Mount Lowe fire road. Turn right (north) and proceed up the fire road. You will begin to notice the unmistakable scars of the 2009 Station Fire. Within the next mile, you pass such viewpoints of yesteryear as Cape of Good Hope; Horseshoe Curve; and, most famous of all, Grand Circular Bridge. There is no bridge here now, just a sharp hairpin turn of the road. After following the slope above Millard Canyon, you round the mountain and turn east high above Grand Canyon, passing through the remains of the rock outcrop once known as Granite Gate. At 6.2 miles, you finally reach

Mount Lowe Trail Camp, nestled in a grove of oaks and firs. The stone wall foundation just east of camp is all that remains of old Mount Lowe Tavern (GPS N34° 13.588' W118° 06.592').

From the trail camp, continue up the fire road, going right (southeast) at a road junction, to the ramada at Inspiration Point (6.6 miles; GPS N34° 13.291' W118° 06.561'). Immediately east of the point is the marked trail dropping into Castle Canyon. Follow this narrow trail as it zigzags steeply down through fir- and oak-shaded Castle Canyon; around the head of Rubio Canyon, where you cross a small creek (which usually has water); and over to Echo Mountain again (8.2 miles). Then descend the Sam Merrill Trail to Altadena.

VARIATION An alternate route between Echo Mountain and Mount Lowe Trail Camp is the old Sunset Trail, signed at both ends as the Sam Merrill Trail. From Echo Mountain, it starts up the crest of the ridge directly to the north; zigzags up and around what was known in Mount Lowe Railway days as Sunset Point; turns east, paralleling the old railway bed about 200 feet above it; and intersects the Mount Lowe fire road about 300 yards south of the trail camp.

To locate the trail from above, follow the fire road 300 yards south from Mount Lowe Trail Camp to a road junction; the trail goes right (west) just south of the junction. This Sunset (or Upper Sam Merrill) Trail is regularly maintained by volunteers from Altadena and other nearby communities. This variation is about the same distance as the regular route.

▪ Hike 19 ECHO MOUNTAIN 🡕 🐕

HIKE LENGTH 5 miles out-and-back; 1,400' elevation gain
DIFFICULTY Moderate
SEASON November–May
MAP Tom Harrison *Angeles Front Country*
PERMIT N/A

▪ FEATURES

If not for the efforts of a handful of public-spirited and sentimental Pasadena and Altadena residents, the Mount Lowe Railway would be all but forgotten today. These people have given freely of their time and effort in

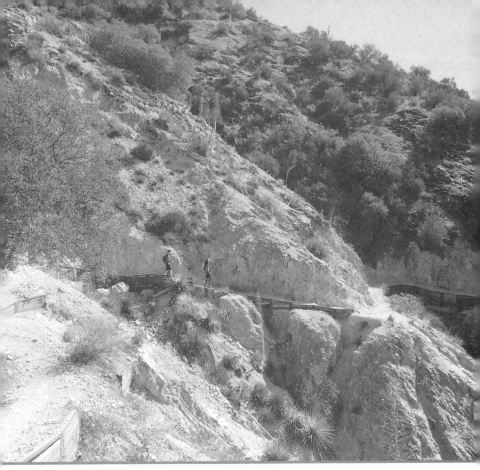

The Echo Mountain Trail is not for the acrophobic.

restorative projects, enabling today's visitor to relive some of this bygone era when cable cars and trolleys climbed high on the mountain.

One of these volunteer efforts was the construction and maintenance of the Sam Merrill Trail from Altadena to Echo Mountain. The trail was built during the 1930s by Charles Warner and the Forest Conservation Club of Pasadena to replace the original, overgrown footpath. During the 1940s it was maintained and improved by Samuel Merrill of Altadena, retired clerk of the Superior Court of Los Angeles. After Merrill's death in 1948, the pathway was named in his honor. Today this trail, one of the most popular in the San Gabriels, is kept in excellent condition by local volunteers.

Back in the early years of the Mount Lowe Railway, Echo Mountain was known as the White City. Perched on top were two hotels—Echo Mountain House and The Chalet—as well as a powerhouse; a machine shop; a dormitory; a reservoir; a small zoo; the Mount Lowe Observatory; and, so it would not be forgotten after dark, the world's most powerful searchlight. All but the searchlight were painted white, clearly visible from the valley below. To reach the White City, tourists were hoisted up the cable incline in white "chariots."

Through a series of fires and windstorms, the White City was destroyed— Echo Mountain House first (1900), then all but the observatory (1905), and finally the observatory itself (1928). The incline was abandoned in 1938.

Only ruins remain today. To commemorate what once was here, a bronze plaque is embedded in cement next to the old incline bull wheel. Among the foundations, Coulter pines and incense cedars, planted by conservation groups in 1941 and 1948, are growing tall.

This trip takes you up the Sam Merrill Trail to Echo Mountain, gives you a guided tour of where once stood the White City, and returns you the same way.

■ DESCRIPTION

From the 210 Freeway in Pasadena, take Exit 26 for Lake Avenue. Go north on Lake Avenue for 3.6 miles to where the street bends left and becomes Loma Alta Drive (GPS N34° 12.236' W118° 07.832'). Find curbside parking near this intersection.

To your right (east), near a large locked gate, is the beginning of the Sam Merrill Trail to Echo Mountain. The first part of the trail crosses the historic Cobb Estate, built by lumberman Charles Cobb in 1918, torn down by the Marx brothers in 1959, acquired on behalf of youth activists to prevent development in 1971, and then donated to the U.S. Forest Service for preservation. Paranormal enthusiasts now call the area the Haunted Forest, and at least two bodies have been found on the property.

Follow the trail east alongside a fence. Where it turns left (north), continue straight ahead and pick up the trail as it crosses Las Flores Canyon and climbs up the east slope of the canyon. After 2.6 zigzagging miles, you reach the ridge behind (north of) Echo Mountain. Here you intersect the old railway bed (see Hike 18). Turn right (south) and follow the railway bed about 100 yards to the Echo Mountain ruins (GPS N34° 12.657' W118° 07.249'). You come first to the commemorative plaque and the old incline bull wheel, embedded in cement. Just beyond, the wall on your left is the foundation of Echo Mountain House, and the pile of concrete rubble ahead is what remains of the incline depot and powerhouse, dynamited by the U.S. Forest Service in 1959. From the steps of Echo Mountain House, you can look directly down the incline bed, descending 1,300 feet into Rubio Canyon. (See Hike 20 for an unmaintained trail down the steep slope.) East of the Echo Mountain House site, 100 feet down the ridge, is the site of The Chalet. Nothing remains of this first hotel. The Mount Lowe Observatory, housing a 13-inch telescope, was located behind Echo Mountain, 0.25 mile up the ridge. Directly below the observatory was the reservoir. After immersing yourself in history and taking in the view, return the way you came.

■ Hike 20 RUBIO CANYON 🡕 🐕 👫

HIKE LENGTH 1.5 miles out-and-back; 200' elevation gain
DIFFICULTY Easy
SEASON November–May
MAP Tom Harrison *Angeles Front Country*
PERMIT N/A

■ FEATURES

Rubio Canyon was once one of the premier scenic attractions of the San Gabriel Mountains, visited by thousands of tourists. For 43 years (1893–1936), Rubio Canyon was an important way station on the Mount Lowe Railway. Tourists rode the winding electric trolley into the canyon, and then climbed aboard the white "chariots" for the ride up the cable incline to Echo

Rubio Pavilion (circa 1894)

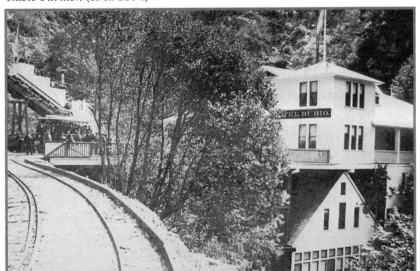

Mountain. Professor Thaddeus S. C. Lowe's elegant Rubio Pavilion stood at the foot of the incline, set amid a forest garden of sycamores, live oaks, ferns, and wildflowers. Radiating up and down the canyon from the edifice were more than a mile of planked walks and rustic stairways, leading through a picturesque setting of ferns, mossy nooks, and miniature waterfalls. All this came to an end in 1909, when a severe thunderstorm sent huge boulders crashing down on the pavilion, demolishing the double-decked structure and causing the only death in all the years of the Mount Lowe operation. From then until the railway's end, Rubio Canyon was nothing but a transfer point for passengers bound for Mount Lowe Tavern.

Today this scene is difficult to visualize. Nothing remains of the magnificent pavilion that once spanned the canyon. The lower end of the incline has been completely eroded, and all the rails have been removed.

In 1998, workers hired by the Rubio Canyon Land and Water Association tried to reroute a water pipe damaged in the 1994 Northridge earthquake. While carving a notch in the steep canyonside, the workers accidentally triggered an avalanche that buried the little waterfalls and cascades under thousands of tons of boulders and debris. The accident embarrassed the U.S. Forest Service, which owns the land, and outraged environmentalists, who demanded that the 100-foot-deep pile of rocks be removed. But federal officials denied responsibility for the cleanup, and the water company claimed that it didn't have the funds to pay for it. Then, in October 2004, a series of strong autumn storms dumped more than 10 inches of rain on the area. In what must have been an awesome display, 50,000 tons of rock and debris were swept away and strewn down the canyon. Old waterfalls were reborn and streams resumed their courses. Of course, there are still scars, and the area retains a raw, unkempt look that will take decades to soften, but Rubio Canyon is on the way to recovery.

■ DESCRIPTION

From the 210 Freeway in Pasadena, take Exit 26 for Lake Avenue. Go north on Lake Avenue 3.0 miles to turn right at Dolores Drive. In 0.4 mile turn right onto Rubio Canyon Road. In 0.3 mile, turn left onto Rubio Crest Drive, then make a quick right onto Rubio Vista Road. Park on the street near the corner of Rubio Vista Road and Pleasantridge Drive near 1342 Rubio Vista Road (GPS N34° 12.180' W118° 07.376').

Take a narrow dirt path between the two houses on the corner, leading north into Rubio Canyon. Just beyond the houses lies the old railway bed that once took passengers to Rubio Pavilion. Proceed along this eroded bed, mostly easygoing but overgrown in spots. The trail hugs a steep drop and is not recommended for those afraid of heights. In 0.5 mile you round a bend to reach footings at the site of Rubio Pavilion. A steep, unmarked use trail climbs left toward Echo Mountain, but we stay right and follow the path down to the canyon bottom. Pick your way among the boulders and debris up the canyon several hundred yards to the base of Moss Grotto and Rock Ribbon Falls (GPS N34° 12.438' W118° 06.990'). Scrambling up the rotten rock is unsafe, and most hikers turn around here.

VARIATION If you don't mind following a steep canyoneer's trail, you can see some of the falls higher in Rubio Canyon. Start up a scree-filled gully to your right. You'll immediately find a trail forking left that leads up a steep slope to above the lower falls, giving you good views of Grand Chasm Falls (GPS N34° 12.472' W118° 06.976'). You may see remains of a stone dam Professor Lowe built above the falls to feed an electrical generator powering Rubio Pavilion.

If you stay in the gully until it becomes rocky and then traverse left under a rock face, you can climb to a shoulder of the ridge called Lunch Spot (GPS N34° 12.470' W118° 06.934'), where you'll have great views of 100-foot-tall Thalehaha Falls.

Experienced canyoneers can make a wonderful descent of Rubio Canyon with 12 rappels. See ropewiki.com for details. A party without adequate skill and gear could get into much trouble here.

VARIATION From Rubio Pavilion, adventurous hikers can follow the use trail up Echo Mountain along the route of the old cable incline, with 1,200 feet of elevation gain over 1 mile. From there, you can descend Echo Mountain via the Sam Merrill Trail (see Hike 19). At a switchback overlooking Rubio Canyon, take an easily missed path on the left that descends back to Rubio Canyon near where you began. This loop is 4 miles with 1,400 feet of elevation gain.

■ Hike 21 EATON CANYON FALLS 🡕 🐕 🧍

HIKE LENGTH 3.5 miles out-and-back; 500' elevation gain

DIFFICULTY Easy

SEASON All year

MAP Tom Harrison *Angeles Front Country*

PERMIT N/A

■ FEATURES

Eaton Canyon Natural Area is a well-known gem at the foot of the San Gabriel Mountains. On a pleasant spring weekend, thousands of people gather at the busy trailhead for a stroll. The Nature Center is full of knowledgeable volunteers who share a passion for the outdoors.

Upstream from the 190-acre park, where the waters of Eaton Canyon have carved a raw groove in the San Gabriel Mountains, you'll discover Eaton Canyon Falls. Impressive only during the wetter half of the year, the falls possesses, as John Muir once put it, "a low sweet voice, singing like a bird." The falls are well worth visiting, especially in the aftermath of a larger

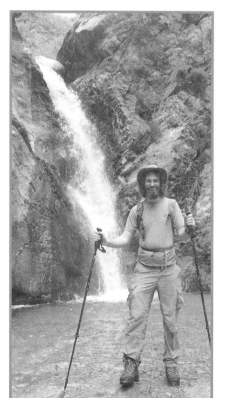

winter storm, if only to witness the power of large (by meager Southern California standards anyway) volumes of falling water. The canyon is named for Judge Benjamin Eaton, who tapped water here for his Fair Oaks Ranch, which is now north Pasadena.

■ DESCRIPTION

From the eastbound 210 Freeway, take Exit 28 for northbound Altadena Drive. (From the westbound 210, take Exit 29A for Sierra Madre and follow the frontage road to Altadena Drive.) Proceed 1.7 miles

The author at Eaton Canyon Falls
KIBY MCDANIEL

to the Nature Center parking on the right, or the nearby overflow area (GPS N34° 10.711' W118° 05.799').

From the parking lot at Eaton Canyon Nature Center, follow the Eaton Canyon Trail upstream. The trail promptly splits—the two branches run parallel and then rejoin before crossing to the east side of the canyon. After crossing the canyon's cobbled bottom, the trail sticks to an elevated stream terrace, passing some beautiful live-oak woods.

At 1.2 miles you rise to meet the Mount Wilson Toll Road bridge over Eaton Canyon. Just before the bridge, veer left onto a narrow track at a sign for Eaton Canyon Falls. The rough path leads up the canyon, crossing the creek eight times. Expect plenty of boulder hopping, and you may get your feet wet if the stream is lively. This is not a place to be when the creek is in flood. Except for a line of alders along part of the stream and some live oaks on terraces just above the reach of floods, the canyon bottom and the precipitous walls are desolate and desertlike. At 1.8 miles, you come to the falls, where the water slides and then free-falls a total of about 35 vertical feet down a narrow chute in the bedrock (GPS N34° 11.803' W118° 06.132').

VARIATION The walk can be shortened to 1.5 miles out-and-back by starting from the lower gate of the Mount Wilson Toll Road on Pinecrest Drive in Altadena (GPS N34° 11.506' W118° 06.327'; see next hike). Make sure to observe the strict parking restrictions in that neighborhood.

■ **Hike 22 HENNINGER FLATS** ↗ 🐕 🚶 ☉ 🏃

HIKE LENGTH 5.5 miles out-and-back; 1,400' elevation gain

DIFFICULTY Moderate

SEASON November–June

MAP Tom Harrison *Angeles Front Country*

PERMIT N/A

■ **FEATURES**

Above Altadena, the scars of the old Mount Wilson Toll Road are clearly visible, zigzagging sharply up the chaparral-covered mountainside from the mouth of Eaton Canyon. A rather conspicuous forested bench is located about a third of the way up. This is Henninger Flats, home of the Los Angeles County Experimental Forestry Nursery.

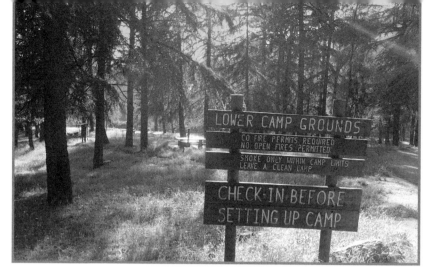

Henninger Flats has many shaded campsites and outstanding nighttime views over the Los Angeles Basin.

The flats have a rich history. They were originally homesteaded by "Captain" William K. Henninger, who grew hay, corn, vegetables, fruit, and melons on his "farm in the clouds." In the early 1900s the flats were leased to the U.S. Forest Service, and under the guidance of Theodore P. Lukens, the first scientific reforestation experiments in California were conducted. Thousands of seedlings from the nursery here were transplanted to fire-blackened slopes all over Southern California.

Since 1928 Henninger Flats and the surrounding slopes have been under the administration of Los Angeles County foresters, who grow thousands of new tree seedlings each year, including knobcone pine, Coulter pine, Canary Island pine, Monterey pine, and Aleppo pine, as well as varieties of cypress, cedar, and sequoia. An administration building with a museum on the ground floor, open to the public on weekends, displays reforestation and historical exhibits, and the county maintains a picnic area and a free first-come, first-served public campground, set amid the shade of tall pines.

Be aware that the route is almost completely shadeless, and during warm weather the hike is best done early in the morning. Bring plenty of water; you may find none available at Henninger.

■ **DESCRIPTION**

From the eastbound 210 Freeway, take Exit 28 for Altadena Drive north. (From westbound 210, take Exit 29A for Sierra Madre and follow the frontage road to Altadena Drive.) Proceed 2.7 miles, then turn right onto Crescent

Drive and immediately right again onto Pinecrest Drive, where you will find the gated trailhead at 2260 Pinecrest Drive (GPS N34° 11.506' W118° 06.327'). Parking is heavily restricted in this area, so carefully observe the signs; you may have to return to Altadena Drive to find parking.

Walk past the locked gate, down across Eaton Canyon, and up the wide old road, zigzagging up steep, chaparral-covered slopes 2.6 miles to Henninger Flats (GPS N34° 11.605' W118° 05.377'). Just inside the shady flats, on both sides of the road, are the picnic area and campground. Straight ahead are the administration building and museum. Behind the museum and to the right are the structures of the county reforestation nursery. A fire lookout tower, formerly atop Castro Peak in the Santa Monicas, stands as a historical exhibit. Return the same way you came.

VARIATIONS From Henninger Flats, you could continue up the toll road to Mount Wilson (see next hike) or follow the Idlehour Trail into upper Eaton Canyon (see Hike 24).

■ Hike 23 MOUNT WILSON TOLL ROAD
↗ 🐐 ⊛ 🏃

HIKE LENGTH 9 miles one-way; 4,500' elevation loss or gain
DIFFICULTY Moderate (downhill) or strenuous (uphill)
SEASON November–June
MAP Tom Harrison *Angeles Front Country*
PERMIT N/A

■ FEATURES

Note: This hike is within the Bobcat Fire Closure Area and is closed at least through April 1, 2022, although it appears to be undamaged. Check with the U.S. Forest Service (fs.usda.gov/angeles) before visiting.

Back in the 1920s, when the age of the automobile arrived in Southern California, the Mount Wilson Toll Road was a favorite of strong-nerved drivers. Narrow, zigzagging, and cliff-hanging much of the way, without side rails, this auto route from Altadena to the summit of Mount Wilson often saw heavy holiday traffic. For those who preferred not to drive themselves, there was the popular Mount Wilson Stage, making the upward grind twice a day—more often when the traffic demanded. Surprisingly, there were few

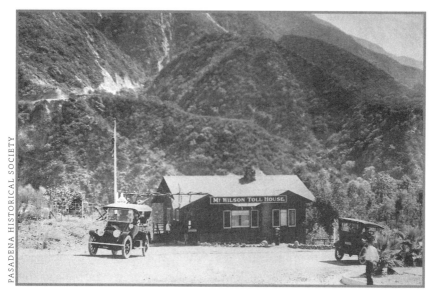

Mount Wilson Toll House (1914)

accidents. Evidently, the obvious dangers served as a cautioning influence. The most amazing episode in the road's long history was the Altadena–Mount Wilson automobile race, held several times during the 1920s. The 9-mile, 4,500-foot, 44-hairpin-turn event makes the more famous Pikes Peak road race pale by comparison. The record for the contest was 22 minutes flat, set in 1922 by Pasadenan Frank Benedict, driving a Paige 6-66.

It was the Pasadena and Mount Wilson Toll Road Company, incorporated in 1889, that first envisioned a road to the mountaintop. Two years later the company completed a 4-foot-wide toll trail to the summit—50 cents per rider, 25 cents per hiker. Not until 1907 was the trail widened to a 10-foot roadway, this to transport the 60-inch telescope to its mountaintop home. In 1912 the toll road was widened to 12 feet to accommodate the 100-inch telescope and was opened to the public, and for the next 24 years it was a popular Sunday drive except among the fainthearted. The end for this historic route came in 1936. Superseded by the new Angeles Crest Highway, it was closed to the public and turned over to the U.S. Forest Service for use as a fire road. So it remains today.

Mount Wilson, home of one of the world's great observatories, is probably the best-known mountain in Southern California. It was named for

Benjamin Wilson, who built the first modern trail to its summit in 1864 (see Hike 34). The first telescope on the peak was the 13-inch refractor of the short-lived Harvard Observatory (1889–1890). Since 1904, the famed Carnegie Observatory has been here, thanks to the enthusiasm and efforts of two farsighted men: astronomer George Ellery Hale and businessman turned philanthropist Andrew Carnegie. From its installation in 1917 until it was surpassed by the 200-incher on Palomar Mountain in 1946, the 100-inch Hooker reflector on Mount Wilson was the world's largest. Today the Mount Wilson observatory is operated on behalf of the Carnegie Institution by the nonprofit Mount Wilson Institute.

In 1948 television came to Mount Wilson in the form of transmitting stations for all seven Los Angeles channels. Mount Wilson's natural flora was supplemented by a man-made forest of antennas, towers, and domes, most of them visible from the valley below. Television not only came but also conquered. In 1964, Metromedia Inc., operators of TV station KTTV, purchased the entire mountaintop from the old Mount Wilson Hotel Company. The rambling old hotel, a fixture on the mountain since 1915 (a previous hotel was built in 1905 and burned in 1913), was torn down, and in its place rose Skyline Park, complete with a pavilion, a children's zoo, and picnic areas. Metromedia deeded the mountaintop to the U.S. Forest Service in 1976. Old-timers would hardly recognize the mountaintop today.

You can tackle the old toll road in two ways. The easier is to have someone drive you to Mount Wilson (19 miles from La Cañada Flintridge), and then hike or mountain bike down. Much more strenuous is to hike up the road from Altadena. Either way, you are rewarded with a close-at-hand view of the abrupt, chaparral-coated south slope of the front range, and you will marvel at the fortitude and backbone of those who once drove this tortuous roadway to the sky. Bring plenty of water, and don't do this hike in warm weather, as much of the route traverses shadeless chaparral.

■ DESCRIPTION

This one-way trip requires a 45-minute shuttle between trailheads. Unless you are using a ride-hailing service, leave one car near the Pinecrest Drive trailhead. From the eastbound 210 Freeway, take Exit 28 for Altadena Drive north. (From the westbound 210, take Exit 29A for Sierra Madre and follow the frontage road to Altadena Drive.) Proceed north on Altadena

Drive for 2.7 miles, then turn right onto Crescent Drive and immediately right again onto Pinecrest Drive, where you will find the gated trailhead at 2260 Pinecrest Drive (GPS N34° 11.506' W118° 06.327'). Parking is heavily restricted in this area, so carefully observe the signs; you may have to return to Altadena Drive to find parking.

To reach the upper trailhead, return to the 210 and continue 8 miles west to the Angeles Crest Highway (Highway 2; Exit 20) in La Cañada Flintridge. Drive 14 miles north and east to Red Box Station and the inter-section of Mount Wilson Road (mile marker 2 LA 38.38). Turn right on Mount Wilson Road and proceed 5 miles to the gate outside Mount Wilson Observatory Skyline Park (GPS N34° 13.498' W118° 03.865'). The top of the Mount Wilson Toll Road is now gated dirt Forest Road 2N45.

From the gate at the top of 2N45/Mount Wilson Toll Road, begin your long switchbacking descent. Watch for signs of the 50-acre 2017 Wilson Fire that threatened the observatory and antenna farm. After 1.0 mile, stay left on the toll road at a fork, where you meet a service road to Mount Harvard and a footpath descending from Skyline Park. This was the site of Martin's Camp from 1891 to 1896, with a wooden dining hall and tent cabins for 40 guests. Little evidence of the camp remains.

At 1.5 miles, stay right at an intersection with the Mount Wilson Trail leading down to Sierra Madre (see Hike 35) or Chantry Flat (see Hike 38). At 5.0 miles, stay left as you pass the Idlehour Trail (see next hike). Con-tinue down through Henninger Flats (6.1 miles; Hike 22), where you can find pleasant camping and picnic grounds shaded beneath an experimental forest. Check in at the Visitor Information Station for a free camping and fire permit, or call ahead (626-794-0675). Drinking water is usually unavailable. After a long, switchbacking descent, cross the bridge at the mouth of Eaton Canyon and arrive at the Pinecrest trailhead.

■ Hike 24 IDLEHOUR TRAIL ↗ 🐕 🚶

HIKE LENGTH 14 miles one-way; 4,100' elevation gain

DIFFICULTY Strenuous

SEASON November–May

MAP Tom Harrison *Angeles Front Country*

PERMIT N/A

■ FEATURES

Few San Gabriel canyons compare with Eaton in ruggedness and inaccessibility. Precipitous sidewalls plunge down from lofty ridges to make this V-shaped gorge in the heart of the front range. A tumbling stream hurries down the length of the chasm, finally to plunge over idyllic Eaton Canyon Falls just above the canyon's mouth. The upper end of the canyon widens into a broad basin under the towering white faces of Mount Markham and San Gabriel Peak.

Trails into Eaton Canyon have always been difficult to build and maintain because of the rugged terrain. The Eaton Falls trail penetrates the lower gorge as far as the first waterfall (Hike 21), beyond which many adventurous hikers have been hurt or killed (the Altadena Rescue Group is called out to Eaton Canyon 30–40 times a year). Well-prepared canyoneers can make a technical descent when the water is not too high; see ropewiki.org for details. You avoid the difficult lower gorge by using the Mount Wilson Toll Road to climb above the canyon and then drop into its gentler upper reaches via the Idlehour Trail.

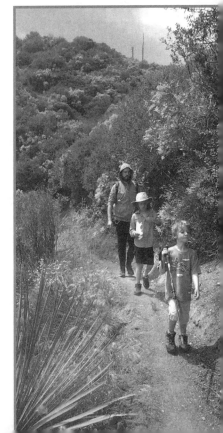

You reach the canyon floor at Idlehour Trail Camp, a secluded spot of unusual natural charm. Here, the creek experiences one of its few serene moods, and a fine forest of oaks, bays, and big-cone Douglas-firs provides cover. In this woodsy haunt once stood Camp Idle Hour, a small trail resort of the Great Hiking Era. The name signified the quiet, restful mood of the place, and throughout its existence (1915–1929), the camp was a favorite of lovers of sylvan seclusion.

The trip is a rather long one, involving much up-and-down, as all

Descending the Idlehour Trail

visits into upper Eaton Canyon must. But it samples some of the most scenic country in the front range. With a short shuttle, your itinerary follows a great loop, dropping into Eaton Canyon from the east and climbing out via the west slope. If a car shuttle is not available, you can retrace your steps, covering just half of the loop. In any event, be in top shape; it's an all-day hike for most people.

■ DESCRIPTION

This trip requires a 2.8-mile car or bicycle shuttle. To leave a getaway vehicle at the Sam Merrill Trailhead, take Exit 26 from the 210 Freeway north for Lake Avenue and drive north for 3.6 miles to where the street bends left and becomes Loma Alta Drive (GPS N34° 12.236' W118° 07.832'). Find curbside parking near this intersection. To reach the start of the trip at the base of the Mount Wilson Toll Road, drive back south on Lake Avenue 1.0 mile, then turn left onto Altadena Drive. In 1.5 miles, turn left onto Crescent Drive, then in 0.1 mile turn right onto Pinecrest Drive, where you will find the gated trailhead at 2260 Pinecrest Drive (GPS N34° 11.506' W118° 06.327'). Parking is heavily restricted in this area, so carefully observe the signs; you may have to return to Altadena Drive to find parking.

Walk around the gate, over the bridge at the mouth of Eaton Canyon, and up the old toll road, passing Henninger Flats at 2.7 miles. At 3.9 miles, look for the Idlehour Trail leading left where the road switchbacks right. Follow the trail over a slight rise and steeply down to Idlehour Trail Camp in Eaton Canyon (5.6 miles; GPS N34° 12.510' W118° 05.049'). The camp, on a bench just east of the stream, is a good picnic or overnight spot, equipped with tables and stoves.

From Idlehour Trail Camp the trail goes upstream, passing the foundations of several old cabins. Much of the path here is washed out, and you must boulder-hop. The pathway crosses the creek, turns sharply left (west), zigzags steeply up and around a ridge, contours into a side canyon (usually a small trickle of water), and continues up to meet a spur of the Mount Lowe fire road, at 9.2 miles. Turn left (southeast) on the spur road to the ramada at Inspiration Point (9.5 miles). Just east of the point is a signed trail dropping down Castle Canyon (see Hike 18). Follow this trail down to Echo Mountain (11.5 miles), and then take the Sam Merrill Trail (see Hike 19) to Lake Avenue in Altadena, downhill all the way.

■ Hike 25 SAN GABRIEL PEAK FROM RED BOX 🡥 🐐

HIKE LENGTH 4 miles out-and-back; 1,400' elevation gain

DIFFICULTY Moderate

SEASON All year

MAP Tom Harrison *Angeles Front Country*

PERMIT N/A

■ FEATURES

Mount Disappointment (5,994') stands high on the crest of the front range, but not quite as high as its next-door summit, San Gabriel Peak. Hence the "disappointment" when some government surveyors lugged their equipment to the top in 1875 and then had to continue to the higher summit to do their surveying.

Aerial view of San Gabriel Peak from the west after a winter snowstorm

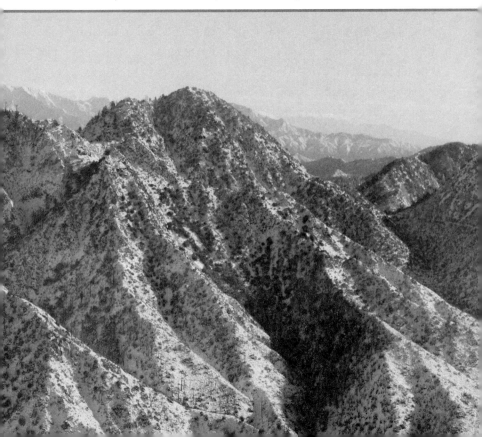

This trip follows the Bill Riley Trail, built by the JPL Hiking Club in 1988, then the upper end of the Mount Disappointment fire road to gain the San Gabriel Peak–Mount Disappointment saddle, and then climbs both peaks. The views from both summits are panoramic. Sadly, the oak, fir, and pine forest that once shaded the upper reaches of both peaks was nearly all burned away in the 2009 Station Fire.

■ DESCRIPTION

Exit the 210 Freeway at Angeles Crest Highway (Highway 2; Exit 20) in La Cañada Flintridge. Drive 14 miles north and east to Red Box Station and the intersection of Mount Wilson Road at mile marker 2 LA 38.38. Turn right on Mount Wilson Road and proceed 0.4 mile to a turnout at the gated Mount Disappointment service road (2N52) on the right (GPS N34° 15.265' W118° 06.126').

Take the San Gabriel Peak Trail, which begins about 50 feet to the left (east) of the fire-road gate. The trail switchbacks up, under a canopy of big-cone Douglas-firs and live oaks, to a junction with the upper section of the Mount Disappointment fire road at 1.2 miles. You begin to encounter evidence of the 2009 Station Fire that becomes more widespread as you near the top. Proceed 200 yards up the fire road to a hairpin turn on the ridgetop. Take the trail left as it drops 50 feet to a fork at the San Gabriel Peak–Mount Disappointment saddle and then climbs the west ridge of San Gabriel Peak to the summit at 1.9 miles (GPS N34° 14.596' W118° 05.918').

On your return, consider following the fire road through the charred remains of the forest that once grew here to the summit of Mount Disappointment, 0.25 mile from the saddle. The top is cluttered with electronic installations and empty buildings dating from the 1950s, when an Army Nike missile station was located here to deter Russian nuclear bombers.

Descend the way you came, or take the fire road all the way down. Either route leads back to your car, but the fire road is a mile longer.

VARIATION With a 2-mile car or bicycle shuttle, you can return to the fork at the San Gabriel–Disappointment saddle and follow the trail south to Markham Saddle and then the fire road east to Eaton Saddle (see Hike 28). This option is 0.5 mile shorter than retracing your steps.

- ## Hike 26 MOUNT LOWE FROM EATON SADDLE 🥾 🐐 🚶

HIKE LENGTH 3 miles out-and-back; 500' elevation gain
DIFFICULTY Easy
SEASON November–June
MAP Tom Harrison *Angeles Front Country*
PERMIT N/A

- ## FEATURES

This is the easy way to do historic Mount Lowe. You start from the back side—the Mount Wilson Road—and contour across the white diorite cliffs of San Gabriel Peak to Markham Saddle. Then climb the gentle north slope of the mountain through fire-thinned chaparral and clusters of small oak trees to the bare summit.

In the early days it was called Oak Mountain, for the groves of splendid live oaks on its upper slopes. By this name it was known when Professor Thaddeus S. C. Lowe and a party of leading Pasadena residents ascended it on horseback in 1892. Lowe was showing his friends his proposed mountain railway, then just beginning construction. One of the party proposed the name Mount Lowe in honor of the man in their midst. The motion was carried by a chorus of ayes, and in the words of publicist and writer G. Wharton James, "There above the clouds, it was named; and it will continue to be so named when every one of the party present at the christening shall have been laid away in Mother Earth; and generations yet unborn shall trace its rugged outlines on their physical geographies and call it Mount Lowe."

Lowe planned to continue his mountain railway to the top and construct a summit hotel, but he ran out of funds after reaching the site of Ye Alpine Tavern, 1,000 feet below. During the years of the Mount Lowe Railway, untold thousands climbed to the top via two well-graded trails from the tavern. On the summit were a small, open observation pavilion and a series of view tubes (iron pipes) pointed at various attractions below.

With the burning of Mount Lowe Tavern in 1936 and the abandonment of the mountain railway, visits to Mount Lowe almost ceased, and the trails and summit paraphernalia fell into decay. Thankfully, Sierra Club volunteers have restored one of the trails and polished and relettered the old view tubes. Old Mount Lowe is again worth visiting.

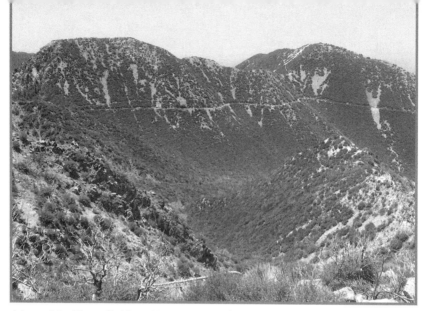

Mount Markham (left) and Mount Lowe (right) from San Gabriel Peak

■ DESCRIPTION

Exit the 210 Freeway at Angeles Crest Highway (Highway 2; Exit 20) in La Cañada Flintridge. Drive 14 miles north and east to Red Box Station and the intersection of Mount Wilson Road at mile marker 2 LA 38.38. Turn right on Mount Wilson Road and proceed 2.4 miles to a roadside parking area at Eaton Saddle (GPS N34° 14.359' W118° 05.606').

Walk past the locked gate onto the Mount Lowe fire road, overlooking the yawning chasm of upper Eaton Canyon. Follow the road as it turns west and contours around the precipitous south face of San Gabriel Peak, tunneling through a nearly vertical cliff at one point. Notice the old guardrails outside the wall, remnants of the airy old Cliff Trail that once joined Mount Lowe Tavern with Mount Wilson. After 0.5 mile you reach Markham Saddle, a V-shaped cleft between San Gabriel Peak and Mount Markham. Here, you leave the road and take an unmarked footpath to the left that leads southwest around the slopes of Mount Markham to the saddle between it and Mount Lowe. You then enter a forest of small oaks as the trail rounds the east slope of Mount Lowe. At 1.2 miles (about 300 yards beyond this last saddle), look for a side trail branching back to your right (west). Leave the main trail (which continues down to Mount Lowe Trail Camp) and walk up the side footpath to the bare summit of Mount Lowe (GPS N34° 13.914' W118° 06.354').

After enjoying the fine vista over the front-range country and pondering the history of this place, return the way you came.

■ Hike 27 MOUNT LOWE TRAIL CAMP FROM EATON SADDLE ◯ 🐕 ⊕ 🏃

HIKE LENGTH 6-mile loop; 1,500' elevation gain
DIFFICULTY Moderate
SEASON November–June
MAP Tom Harrison *Angeles Front Country*
PERMIT N/A

■ FEATURES

This loop trip takes you completely around Mount Lowe and visits secluded Mount Lowe Trail Camp, once the location of famed Mount Lowe Tavern (see Hike 18). Most of the hike is via easy-graded fire road, but about 2 miles are on the historic, oak-shaded Mount Lowe East Trail, recently reworked into good condition. You are rewarded en route with superb vistas down into Eaton Canyon and fire-ravaged Bear and Grand Canyons and, if the atmosphere is clear, down the south slope of the front range to the sprawling San Gabriel Valley.

■ DESCRIPTION

Exit the 210 Freeway at Angeles Crest Highway (Highway 2; Exit 20) in La Cañada Flintridge. Drive 14 miles north and east to Red Box Station and the intersection of Mount Wilson Road at mile marker 2 LA 38.38. Turn right on Mount Wilson Road and proceed 2.4 miles to a roadside parking area at Eaton Saddle (GPS N34° 14.359' W118° 05.606').

Walk past the locked gate and follow the Mount Lowe fire road to Markham Saddle at 0.5 mile, and then turn left on the Mount Lowe East Trail to the saddle between Mounts Markham and Lowe (see Hike 26). Continue on the trail past a junction with the Mount Lowe West Trail (1.3 miles) through a shady oak forest around the east shoulder of Mount Lowe, and then down around the south slope via switchbacks to a badly eroded firebreak. The trail crosses the firebreak and continues zigzagging down to the Mount Lowe fire road. Follow it south 100 yards to meet the Inspiration Point spur road at a five-way junction (2.6 miles), and then right about 300 yards to Mount Lowe Trail Camp (2.8 miles, GPS N34° 13.588' W118° 06.592'). Here, under oaks and firs, there are tables, stoves, restrooms, and a spring-fed cistern (treat the water before drinking). The stone foundation adjacent to the camp is all that remains of old Mount Lowe Tavern, once the scene of much merrymaking.

To return, follow a steep trail from the camp up a gully to Mount Lowe Road. On the far side of the road, pick up the signed Mount Lowe West Trail to complete a circle around the mountain. Consider a short detour to the summit before rejoining the Mount Lowe East Trail at 4.6 miles and following it back to Markham Saddle.

■ Hike 28 SAN GABRIEL PEAK FROM EATON SADDLE

HIKE LENGTH 3 miles out-and-back; 1,000' elevation gain
DIFFICULTY Moderate
SEASON November–June
MAP Tom Harrison *Angeles Front Country*
PERMIT N/A

■ FEATURES

Pyramidal San Gabriel Peak towers high on the crest of the front range. From its 6,161-foot summit, you get an unmatched 360-degree panorama

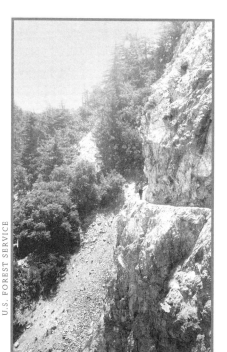

across the wrinkled San Gabriel Mountains, with the front range in the foreground, laced as it is with paved highways, fire roads, trails, firebreaks, and assorted paraphernalia of mankind. The vista is good because the top is tall, small, and apical. You get that airy, top-of-the-world feeling, as you do on nearby Strawberry Peak (see Hike 32).

Famous Cliff Trail between Eaton Saddle and Markham Saddle, now bypassed by Mueller Tunnel

U.S. FOREST SERVICE

There are days when you look down upon canyon-ascending arms of smog rising from the vast megalopolis dimly visible to the south. There are other days when billowing clouds swirl around you, playing hide-and-seek with nearby peaks. And there are those crisp winter and spring days when the sky has been washed clean by a storm and you can see half of Southern California spread out in stark beauty; these are the days to climb San Gabriel Peak.

This climb is short in distance, but the trail is steep and narrow in spots.

■ DESCRIPTION

Exit the 210 Freeway at Angeles Crest Highway (Highway 2; Exit 20) in La Cañada Flintridge. Drive 14 miles north and east to Red Box Station and the intersection of Mount Wilson Road at mile marker 2 LA 38.38. Turn right on Mount Wilson Road and proceed 2.4 miles to a roadside parking area at Eaton Saddle (GPS N34° 14.359' W118° 05.606').

Walk past the locked gate and across the rugged south face of San Gabriel Peak via the Mount Lowe fire road 0.5 mile to Markham Saddle. At the saddle, just beyond the water tank, turn sharply right (north) and pick up an unmarked trail leading up the mountainside. Follow the trail up one switchback, and then across the west slope of San Gabriel Peak to the high saddle between Mount Disappointment and San Gabriel Peak, 1.1 miles from the start. At the saddle, turn right (east) and follow the trail to the top (GPS N34° 14.596' W118° 05.918').

After enjoying your eagle's-eye view, return the way you came. Do not try to descend directly down the ridge (southeast) to Eaton Saddle—the footing is unstable and the chaparral is thick and thorny.

VARIATION From Markham Saddle, you can make a side trip to the dramatic Mount Markham (5,742'). Follow the Mount Lowe trail southwest to another saddle on the ridge between Mounts Lowe and Markham. Turn sharply left and follow a climbers' trail up to the summit of Markham. This variation adds 1.1 miles each way and 500 feet of climbing. Retrace your steps, or take the 0.4-mile excursion to Mount Lowe to make a peak bagger's extravaganza. Mount Markham was named by Professor Lowe in honor of his friend and Pasadena neighbor Henry Markham, governor of California from 1891 to 1895.

▪ Hike 29 BEAR CANYON TRAVERSE 🥾 🐕 🚶

HIKE LENGTH 8 miles one-way; 2,700' elevation loss, 800' elevation gain
DIFFICULTY Moderate
SEASON November–June
MAP Tom Harrison *Angeles Front Country*
PERMIT Post Adventure Pass at Switzer, or park outside fee area.

▪ FEATURES

This trip is a long walk through some of the most scenic parts of the front-range country. The first 8 miles are all downhill, and the last 2 miles are uphill. You may especially enjoy the descent of Bear Canyon to the middle gorge of the Arroyo Seco via the old Tom Sloan Trail, a historic footpath that once joined two of the most popular resorts in the mountains—Mount Lowe Tavern and Switzer's. With the demise of the tavern in 1936, the trail fell into disuse, but it is currently completely passable.

▪ DESCRIPTION

This trip requires a 6-mile shuttle. Leave one vehicle at the Switzer Picnic area. To get here from the 210 Freeway in La Cañada Flintridge, take the Angeles Crest Highway (Highway 2; Exit 20) 10 miles north and east to the Switzer Picnic Area (mile marker 2 LA 34.2). Drive 0.5 mile down the paved access road to the parking lot next to the picnic area, where the road makes a hairpin turn, and leave a vehicle here (GPS N34° 15.969' W118° 08.718'). Drive your other vehicle to Eaton Saddle by returning to the Angeles Crest Highway and continuing east 4 miles to Red Box Station. Turn right on Mount Wilson Road and proceed 2.4 miles to a roadside parking area at Eaton Saddle (GPS N34° 14.359' W118° 05.606'). If you wish to use a bicycle shuttle instead, consider doing the hike in reverse so your bike ride is downhill.

Walk past the locked gate at Eaton Saddle, following the Mount Lowe fire road across the face of San Gabriel Peak to Markham Saddle and then on down the road until it reaches the top of Mount Lowe's long west ridge, 1.8 miles from the start. Here, the road switches back eastward. Leave the road and proceed down the obvious but unmarked trail on the right (north) side of the ridge to Tom Sloan Saddle at 3.0 miles. From the saddle, follow the old Tom Sloan Trail as it drops northwest down into Bear Canyon. At 3.8 miles, you reach the canyon floor, a beautiful spot shaded by big-cone Douglas-firs.

The foundations you see are all that remains of several old cabins, abandoned after a fire many years ago. Continue down Bear Canyon, following the streamside trail or boulder-hopping where the trail has been washed out, to Bear Canyon Trail Camp at 4.8 miles (GPS N34° 14.649' W118° 08.386'), located on a shaded bench on the south side of the creek. This is a perfect lunch stop, as it lies about halfway on your trip, or a good place to spend the night.

Continue downcanyon on lightly maintained trail to the junction with the Arroyo Seco. The trail veers north past delightful pools and cascades of the middle gorge to a junction with the Switzer Falls Spur at 6.6 miles. The 0.2-mile side trip to the falls is worthwhile if the water is flowing well (see Hike 13). However, our hike climbs on the main trail up to a junction with the Gabrielino Trail at 6.8 miles. Turn right (north) and follow the well-beaten footpath through the former Commodore Switzer Trail Camp at 7.1 miles and on to Switzer Picnic Area.

VARIATION You can avoid the car shuttle by making an out-and-back trip from Switzer Picnic Area to Bear Canyon Trail Camp. This scenic trip is 6.5 miles with 1,300 feet of elevation gain total.

■ Hike 30 JONES PEAK 🥾 🐕

HIKE LENGTH 6 miles out-and-back; 2,300' elevation gain
DIFFICULTY Moderate
SEASON November–May
MAP Tom Harrison *Angeles Front Country*
PERMIT N/A

■ FEATURES

Towering directly over the foothill community of Sierra Madre, 3,375-foot Jones Peak divides the watersheds of the Little Santa Anita Canyon (see Hikes 35 and 36) to the east, and rugged, steep, narrow Bailey Canyon, where this trip originates.

The canyon was homesteaded in 1875 by R. J. Bailey, but he soon sold it, and the property passed through a succession of title holders. Today it is owned by the city of Sierra Madre, which operates it as Bailey Canyon Park. Jones Peak was named for the first mayor of Sierra Madre, C. W. Jones, who served from 1907 to 1914 and was a longtime resident of the town, living to the age of 99 before his death in 1967.

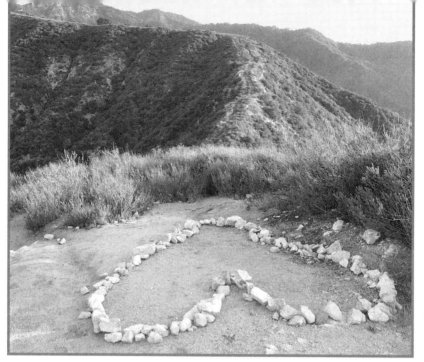

Rock art atop Jones Peak

Most of the trail is shadeless and, if the day is sunny, hot. Do it early in the morning or on a cool winter or spring day, and be prepared for the final, steep scramble to the peak.

■ DESCRIPTION

From the 210 Freeway in Arcadia, take Exit 31 (Baldwin Avenue). Drive 1.6 miles north to turn left on Carter Avenue. Proceed 0.5 mile west to reach the day-use parking lot at Bailey Canyon Park (GPS N34° 10.263' W118° 03.686').

This trip has a convoluted start but soon becomes well-defined. From the northwest corner of the parking lot, head west past the picnic area and exit through a turnstile onto a paved road. Go north toward the canyon, clearly visible ahead. The road soon turns to dirt and becomes a footpath. Pass a bridge on the right leading to an undermaintained nature trail. Continue straight to another junction at 0.4 mile. The left fork goes 0.2 mile to Bailey Falls, worth a side trip only when the creek is running strong. Our trip bears right as the trail begins to head uphill. The trail switchbacks steeply up the east wall of the canyon, passing two benches with great views. At 2.1 miles you enter the welcome shade of a live oak forest near the ruins of a small cabin, a nice spot for a break. Continue up the trail as it climbs another

700 feet to Jones Saddle just north of the peak, at 3.0 miles. From here, it's a short but steep scramble up to the top (GPS N34° 11.188' W118° 03.167'). If it's a clear day, you are rewarded with a spectacular vista of the San Gabriel Valley; downtown Los Angeles; and, if it's exceptionally clear, Catalina. Below, to the east, you look down on the Mount Wilson Trail and Little Santa Anita Canyon. Return the way you came, taking care to watch your footing on the descent.

VARIATIONS From Jones Saddle, a footpath continues north up the ridgeline. You could follow it all the way over Hastings Peak to reach the Mount Wilson Toll Road beneath Yale Mountain in 1.5 miles and then continue to Mount Wilson or Henninger Flats. For a shorter loop, go just 0.1 mile and then turn right onto the signed Connector Trail, which quickly begins to descend steeply into Little Santa Anita Canyon, reaching the Mount Wilson Trail at the bottom in 0.8 mile. Turn right and hike downhill past First Water and back to Mira Monte Avenue in Sierra Madre in another 3 miles. Close the loop in less than a mile on foot by turning right (west) on Mira Monte, jogging right on Auburn Avenue, and turning left on Carter Avenue for a total trip distance of 8 miles.

The most direct descent from Jones Peak is via Bastard Ridge, a steep and severely eroded firebreak on the southeast ridge, reaching a bench (GPS N34° 10.673' W118° 02.796') and continuing down to the Old Mount Wilson Trail just beyond at the mouth of Little Santa Anita Canyon (GPS N34° 10.621' W118° 02.701'), 1.0 mile from the peak. Follow the trail 0.9 mile down to the trailhead on Mira Monte.

■ Hike 31 JOSEPHINE PEAK 🏃 🐕 ⊛

HIKE LENGTH 8 miles out-and-back; 1,900' elevation gain
DIFFICULTY Moderate
SEASON All year
MAP Tom Harrison *Angeles Front Country*
PERMIT N/A

■ FEATURES

Josephine Peak—at 5,558 feet, the high point of the prominent spur extending 2 miles west from Strawberry Peak—offers superb views of the Big Tujunga watershed. A well-graded fire road climbs 4 miles from the Angeles Forest Highway to the fire lookout on the summit. This makes for a pleasant stroll when the weather is mild. Don't try it on a hot day; except for a few forested spots near the top, the route is devoid of shade. An option, if you are in top physical condition, is to climb both Josephine and Strawberry Peaks by this approach, descending the same way or via Colby Canyon.

The origin of the name Josephine is obscure. As early as 1889 there was a Josephine Gold Mine in the upper Big Tujunga. Several authorities believe that the peak was named for the wife of J. B. Lippencott, a U.S. Geological Survey employee who used the summit as a triangulation point while mapping the mountains in 1894. Another source claims that it was named for the daughter of Phil Begue, one of the area's early forest rangers. The fire lookout, erected in 1937, burned down in the 1975 Mill Fire. Josephine burned again in the 2009 Station Fire but has recovered and is an enjoyable hike.

■ DESCRIPTION

Exit the 210 Freeway at Angeles Crest Highway (Highway 2; Exit 20) in La Cañada Flintridge. Drive 9.4 miles north to the junction with the Angeles Forest Highway at mile marker 33.80, where you can park on the shoulder or at the Clear Creek Information Station across the road (GPS N34° 16.217' W118° 09.176').

The Josephine fire road begins on the east side of the Angeles Forest Highway about 50 yards north of the junction. Walk past the locked gate up the road as it climbs the ridge dividing Colby Canyon from Clear Creek and zigzags to the crest of Josephine's east ridge at 2.4 miles. Here, a fire road goes

Josephine Peak's rocky south face seen from Hoyt Mountain

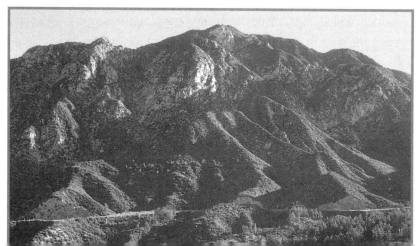

right (east) to Josephine Saddle and Strawberry Peak (see Hike 32) and left (west) to Josephine Peak. Go left, following the road through oaks and firs on the north side of the ridge to the concrete foundation of the summit lookout at 3.9 miles (GPS N34° 17.137' W118° 09.235'). Return by the same route.

VARIATION If you can arrange a 1-mile car or bicycle shuttle, descend to Josephine Saddle and down the old Colby Canyon Trail to the Angeles Crest Highway (see Hike 32). This attractive option is also 8 miles and 1,900 feet of elevation gain. Walking back on the shoulder of the busy highway would be unappealing.

■ Hike 32 STRAWBERRY PEAK ↗

HIKE LENGTH 7 miles out-and-back; 2,600' elevation gain
DIFFICULTY Moderate
SEASON All year
MAP Tom Harrison *Angeles Front Country*
PERMIT N/A

■ FEATURES

Strawberry Peak, a lumpy mass of granite rising 6,164 feet above sea level, is the highest of all the summits of the San Gabriel front range. Looming far above the Angeles Crest Highway between the Arroyo Seco and Big Tujunga watersheds, its airy crown commands a sweeping vista over mountain and lowland. The mountain was severely burned in the 2009 Station Fire, but the trail has been repaired.

Strawberry is the only peak in the front range whose ascent involves more than a plodding walk up. Its nearly vertical upper ramparts give you a taste of the alpinist's exhilaration, and once on top you'll really know that you've climbed a mountain. There, with slopes tapering precipitously on all sides, you get that top-of-the-world feeling. Many hikers consider it the "fun" peak of the San Gabriels.

The peak was labeled by wags at Switzer's Camp back in the 1880s; they thought it resembled a strawberry standing on its stem. It has been a popular climb as long as modern man has trod the San Gabriels. During the Great Hiking Era (1895–1938), backpackers chugging over the well-beaten trail between Switzer's and Colby's often made the airy side trip to take in the rewarding summit panorama. It is just as frequented today. Every fair-weather weekend finds climbers by the scores testing their stamina and skills on its steep granite spine.

In March 1909, Strawberry Peak garnered national attention when a gas balloon and gondola carrying six passengers over Tournament Park in Pasadena was swept by violent gusts into storm clouds over the San Gabriel Mountains. After being tossed as high as 14,000 feet, the balloon descended in whiteout conditions and crash-landed just below Strawberry's snow-covered summit—its gondola coming to rest just 10 feet from a vertical precipice. Nearly three days later, a telephone call from Switzer's Camp brought news to the world below that the riders had survived.

The climb is not particularly difficult for those in good physical condition who have experience on Class 3 rock. Using proper caution—testing hand- and footholds and moving slowly—you should have little trouble if you follow the route indicated by the green arrows painted on boulders. Take extra care on the descent, for that is when most accidents occur.

■ DESCRIPTION

Exit the 210 Freeway at Angeles Crest Highway (Highway 2; Exit 20) in La Cañada Flintridge. Drive 10.2 miles north on Highway 2 to the Colby Canyon trailhead at an unpaved turnout on the left at mile marker 34.55 (GPS N34° 16.193' W118° 08.435').

Proceed up the Colby Canyon Trail, which starts on the left (west) side of the creek. This trail is one of the historic pathways of the range. The trail follows the creek for 0.25 mile, and then climbs steeply up the right side to bypass several small waterfalls where the canyon narrows. You then drop back into the shady, alder-filled upper canyon before switchbacking up through thorny chaparral to Josephine Saddle, 2.1 miles from the highway. Here, you meet the Strawberry Spur of the Josephine fire road.

From Josephine Saddle, the old Colby Canyon Trail winds eastward, around the north flank of Strawberry Peak and down to Strawberry Meadow (see next hike). Do *not* take this trail; instead climb eastward up a steep climbers' path that ascends the crest of the ridge. About 0.25 mile above Josephine Saddle you must negotiate a rocky section of about 75 vertical feet; take care to stay on the trail because getting off route takes you across dangerously crumbling rock. Continue along the ridgecrest to the base of Strawberry Peak's imposing granite summit block. Here, the faint-hearted will turn back; the route looks more difficult than it actually is and has some exposure. Follow the faded green arrows painted at intervals on the rock face, gripping firmly and testing hand- and footholds, to the final summit ridge, and then scramble a hundred feet to the top (3.4 miles; GPS N34° 17.009' W118° 07.227'). Be careful as you descend the same way.

VARIATION You can traverse Strawberry Peak and descend to Red Box to avoid retracing your airy route. Follow an unmaintained but usually good trail east and south to a saddle between Strawberry and Mount Lawlor, where you meet a maintained trail. Turn right and follow it down to Red Box. This trip requires a 3.8-mile car or bicycle shuttle to avoid walking on the shoulder of the busy Angeles Crest Highway. This variation is also 7 miles with 2,600 feet of elevation gain.

From the Strawberry–Lawlor Saddle, you could also circle north on good trail to return to Josephine Saddle, passing a potential campsite at a lovely flat beneath Strawberry's imposing north face. This more demanding loop is 12 miles with 3,500 feet of elevation gain.

■ Hike 33 STRAWBERRY MEADOW 🥾 🐕 ⊕ 🏃

HIKE LENGTH 9 miles out-and-back; 1,600' elevation gain
DIFFICULTY Moderate
SEASON All year
MAP Tom Harrison *Angeles Front Country*
PERMIT Post Adventure Pass, or park on highway outside fee area.

■ FEATURES

The back side of Strawberry Peak holds pleasant surprises. Close under granite cliffs and boulder-stacked ridges, springs seep cold water, and little meadows sprout tall grasses. In the protective shade of the great mountain, forest and chaparral intermingle and grow lush and green. Here, just across the ridge from the busy Angeles Crest Highway, away from ranger stations, public campgrounds, and the assorted miscellany that accompanies civilization, you savor a small touch of wilderness.

This delightful trail trip takes you over the mountain from Red Box to Strawberry Meadow, three small meadows below the great north cliff of

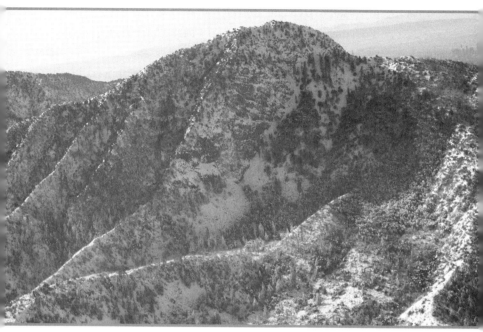

The north face of Strawberry Peak

Strawberry Peak. You pass alternately through clusters of dense chaparral—scrub oak, manzanita, snowbrush, and mountain mahogany—and a varied forest of live oaks, big-cone Douglas-firs, and Jeffrey and Coulter pines. This area burned in the 2009 Station Fire, but the chaparral has made a vigorous recovery. Mountain bikers have beautifully restored the trail. Bring lunch and a good book; you'll want to stay awhile.

■ DESCRIPTION

Exit the 210 Freeway at Angeles Crest Highway (Highway 2; Exit 20) in La Cañada Flintridge. Drive 14 miles north and east to Red Box Station (mile marker 2 LA 38.38, at the intersection of Mount Wilson Road). Park in the lot for the ranger station or picnic ground (GPS N34° 15.530' W118° 06.258').

Cross the Angeles Crest Highway and follow it northeast about 50 yards to the beginning of the abandoned Barley Flats fire road, now a trail. Follow the road 0.8 mile until it becomes severely overgrown, and then turn left and follow good trail up to the ridge and around the mountain to the saddle between Mount Lawlor and Strawberry Peak at 2.3 miles.

From the saddle, continue on the trail as it gently descends around the east and northeast slopes of Strawberry Peak. You pass through alternate stretches of chaparral on sun-exposed slopes and forest on shady north faces. At 4.2 miles, you reach a signed junction with a trail leading north to the private Colby Ranch. Our trip stays left and climbs over a bouldery ridge to the westernmost and largest clearing of Strawberry Meadow, right beneath the towering granite cliffs and a handful of surviving Coulter pines (4.8 miles; GPS N34° 17.327' W118° 06.962'). You could spend a pleasant night here, but be sure to bring your own water.

Return the way you came.

VARIATION With a 4-mile car or bicycle shuttle, you can continue west on the Colby Canyon Trail. Contour around Strawberry Peak to Josephine Saddle at 2 miles, and then follow the trail another 2 miles down to the Colby Canyon Trailhead at mile marker 34.55 on the Angeles Crest Highway. This trip is 9 miles with 1,200 feet of elevation gain.

■ Hike 34 ORCHARD CAMP 🡕 🐕 ❂ 🚶

HIKE LENGTH 7 miles out-and-back; 2,000' elevation gain
DIFFICULTY Moderate
SEASON November–May
MAP Tom Harrison *Angeles Front Country*
PERMIT N/A

■ FEATURES

Note: This hike is within the Bobcat Fire Closure Area and is closed at least through April 1, 2022, although it appears to be undamaged. Check with the U.S. Forest Service (fs.usda.gov/angeles) before visiting.

Beautiful Little Santa Anita Canyon is steeped in history. Ages before the arrival of the white man, Gabrielino Indians forged a rough footpath up the canyon and on to Mount Wilson. Its namesake, Benjamin Wilson, proprietor of the Lake Vineyard Rancho in what is now San Marino and a prominent Southern California resident, built the first modern trail into the San Gabriels up this canyon in 1864 to obtain timber from the mountaintop. In 1889, the Harvard University telescope was toted up this trail piece by piece on its way to occupy the first observatory on Mount Wilson.

In a secluded glen, shaded by giant canyon oaks and big-cone Douglas-firs near the head of the main canyon, Don Benito—as Wilson was known to his many California friends—built his Halfway House in 1864. This original Halfway House, so named because it was midway between Sierra Madre and Mount Wilson, was a construction camp for the original Mount Wilson Trail. Later it was homesteaded by two colorful mountaineers, George Aiken and George Islip, who planted a small grove of apple, cherry, plum, and chestnut trees. With the maturing of these trees, the place became known as Orchard Camp. Around 1890 James McNally made Orchard Camp into a trail resort, and for 50 years this hostelry, under a succession of owners, was one of the most popular in the range. Its peak year was 1911, when more than 40,000 people signed the camp register. Orchard Camp was abandoned in 1940. Today the buildings and tents are gone, but the enchanting streamside spot still holds its appeal.

Most of Little Santa Anita Canyon lies within the Sierra Madre Historical Wilderness Area, owned by the City of Sierra Madre. For years, Ambrose Zaro, "the grand old man" of the trail, almost single-handedly maintained it. His death in March 1990 was mourned by all Mount Wilson Trail hikers. The Mount Wilson Trail Race Committee now keeps the trail in admirable condition under the leadership of Charlie Bell.

Our pleasant trail trip follows this historic footpath from Sierra Madre to old Orchard Camp and back. Take along a picnic lunch and a camera; you'll be so delighted by the woodsy charm of Orchard Camp that you'll want to stay awhile.

■ DESCRIPTION

From the 210 Freeway in Arcadia, take Exit 31 for Baldwin Avenue. Go north 1.5 miles on Baldwin, then turn right on Mira Monte Avenue. Go two blocks east on Mira Monte to reach the Mount Wilson Trailhead on the left (GPS N34° 10.181' W118° 02.952').

Proceed about 150 yards up Mount Wilson Trail Drive to the beginning of the Mount Wilson Trail, marked by a large wooden sign on the left. Follow the trail alongside some private homes up to the ridgetop road, where the main footpath begins. Proceed up the trail as it climbs steadily along the west slope of the canyon, far above the stream. At 0.9 mile, come to your first junction. The Old Mount Wilson Trail stays right and hangs on a dramatic cliff. Those who dislike heights might prefer Charlie's New Trail, which switchbacks up to bypass the cliff before rejoining the main trail. The trail, which opened in 2019, is named for Charlie Bell, who has spent more than three decades maintaining the Old Mount Wilson Trail.

In 1.5 miles you reach another junction. The fork on the right drops to the creek at a popular spot known as First Water, then continues up the stream to the site of the old Quarterway House before climbing up Lost Canyon to rejoin the main trail. This trip continues straight on the main trail, staying high above the stream. Round a ridge and enter the welcome shade of a live oak forest, passing the Connector Trail on the left coming down from Jones Peak. Just beyond is a spur on the right leading to a heliport with excellent views. The trail climbs steadily and then drops to the small creek trickling down from Decker Spring. Beyond, you climb steeply and then contour through cool forest to Orchard Camp, located on a bench shaded by oaks and big-cone Douglas-firs just above the sparkling creek (3.7 miles; GPS N34° 11.939' W118° 03.206'). The huge canyon live oak that had graced this site for some 1,500 years finally toppled on Christmas Day 2017. Return the way you came.

VARIATION Families or youth groups looking for a shorter trip might turn around at First Water. This option is 3 miles and 1,000 feet of elevation gain out-and-back.

■ Hike 35 MOUNT WILSON VIA OLD MOUNT WILSON TRAIL 🡕 🐕 🚶 🚶

HIKE LENGTH 7 miles one-way; 4,500' elevation gain
DIFFICULTY Strenuous (uphill); moderate (downhill)
SEASON November–May
MAP Tom Harrison Angeles Front Country
PERMIT Post Adventure Pass at upper trailhead.

■ FEATURES

Note: This hike is within the Bobcat Fire Closure Area and is closed at least through April 1, 2022, although it appears to be undamaged. Check with the U.S. Forest Service (fs.usda.gov/angeles) before visiting.

This original trail up Mount Wilson—forged by Benjamin Wilson in 1864—has, over the years, been one of the premier attractions in the

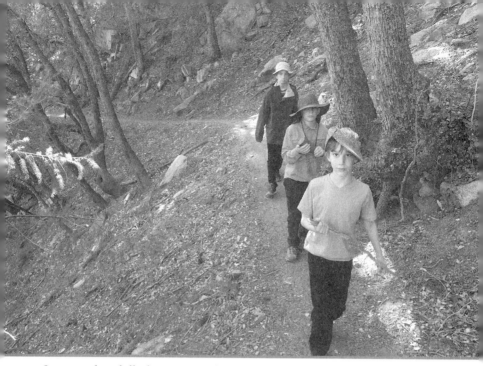

One-way downhill, the Mount Wilson Trail is a good adventure for energetic kids. Uphill is a demanding workout for adults.

range. No trail in the range has a richer heritage. (Its early history, an integral part of the Little Santa Anita Canyon story, is told in the previous hike.) During the Great Hiking Era (1895–1938), the dusty pathway vibrated under the tramp of boots and the pounding of hooves on every fair-weather weekend. Each Saturday morning, hundreds would disembark from the red Pacific Electric trolley cars in Sierra Madre, knapsacks slung over their shoulders, and ramble up the crowded footpath to the mountaintop resorts. Sunday afternoon, often weary and footsore, the hikers would emerge from the mountains to find the big red cars waiting, ready for the homeward journey.

With the end of the hiking era and the distraction of World War II, the old Mount Wilson Trail fell into years of disuse. Gradually it became overgrown and badly eroded in spots. In 1953 UNSAFE TO TRAVEL signs were posted at both ends of the historic pathway. Fortunately, a group of Sierra Madre volunteers, led by Bill Wark, spent many weekends restoring the trail, and it was reopened in 1960. Ambrose Zaro maintained the trail for 30 years before his death in 1990. The Mount Wilson Trail Race Committee now keeps the trail in admirable condition under the leadership of Charlie Bell.

■ DESCRIPTION

This trip requires a 1-hour car shuttle. For an uphill trip, leave your get-away vehicle at the Skyline Park Trailhead at the top of the Mount Wilson Trail. From the 210 Freeway in La Cañada Flintridge, drive 14 miles north and east on Highway 2 to Red Box Station and the intersection of Mount Wilson Road at mile marker 2 LA 38.38. Turn right on Mount Wilson Road and proceed 4 miles to the parking lot at the end of the road (GPS N34° 13.379' W118° 03.772'). To reach the start of the hike, return to the 210 and drive east 10 miles, then take Exit 31 (Baldwin Avenue). Go north 1.5 miles, then turn right on Mira Monte Avenue. Go two blocks east to reach the Mount Wilson Trailhead on the left (GPS N34° 10.181' W118° 02.952'). Be sure to turn your wheels toward the curb (if facing downhill) or away from the curb (if facing uphill) at the trailhead, as local law requires, to prevent your car from rolling into traffic; Sierra Madre aggressively tickets violators.

Walk about 150 yards up Mount Wilson Trail Drive to the beginning of the trail, marked by a large wooden sign. Then follow the trail to Orchard Camp at 3.5 miles (see previous hike). This is the last dependable water source; as always, purify it before drinking. Follow the trail as it climbs steeply through chaparral, canyon live oaks, and big-cone Douglas-firs up the west slope of Little Santa Anita Canyon. The trail crosses the canyon near its head and switches back eastward to the firebreak atop the ridge separating Little Santa Anita from Winter Creek. Here, at 5.2 miles, you intersect the Winter Creek Trail (see Hike 38). Turn left (west) and continue up the trail as it zigzags steeply up to the Mount Wilson Toll Road at 5.8 miles. Turn right and follow the old toll road through an open forest. At 6.4 miles, reach the Wilson–Harvard saddle, once the site of Martin's Camp. Here, you can pick up a shortcut trail up to the parking area at Skyline Park. If you are doing this hike in reverse, beware that the sign at the upper trailhead is missing.

■ Hike 36 STURTEVANT FALLS 🥾 🐕 🚶

HIKE LENGTH 3.3 miles out-and-back; 600' elevation gain
DIFFICULTY Easy
SEASON November–June
MAP Tom Harrison *Angeles Front Country*
PERMIT Post Adventure Pass, or park on road outside fee area.

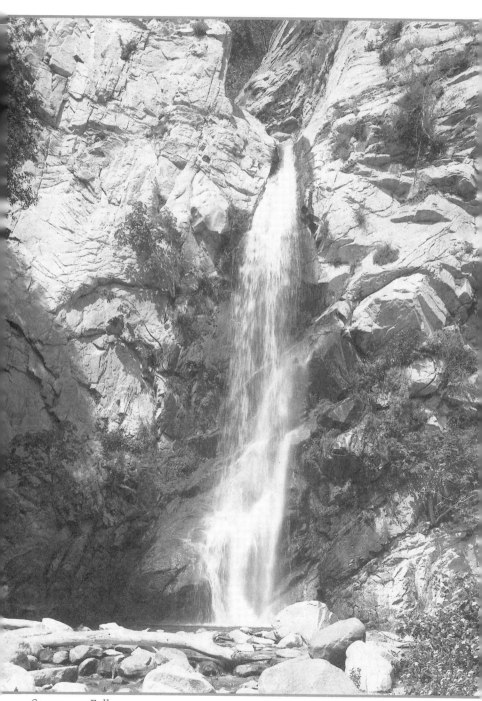

Sturtevant Falls

JOHN W. ROBINSON

■ FEATURES

Note: This hike is within the Bobcat Fire Closure Area and is closed at least through April 1, 2022. Parts of Big Santa Anita Canyon burned severely. Check with the U.S. Forest Service (fs.usda.gov/angeles) before visiting.

Although there are many cascades and small water drops in Big Santa Anita, Sturtevant Falls is the most impressive waterfall in the canyon. Its silver spray plunges 50 feet into a shallow, rock-ribbed pool, shaded by alders and oaks. En route you pass through a beautiful grove of oaks and ferns at the site of old Fern Lodge. In spring, there are fine displays of wildflowers, namely prickly phlox and sticky monkey flower.

This is a short, leisurely stroll from Chantry Flat, a good beginner's hike. You can combine the trip with a picnic under the oaks at Chantry Flat, which has stoves, tables, and water.

■ DESCRIPTION

From the 210 Freeway in Arcadia, take Exit 32 for Santa Anita Avenue and go north 5 miles to the parking lots at Chantry Flat (GPS N34° 11.734' W118° 01.347'), passing a gate open 6 a.m.–8 p.m. The popular trailhead fills early on weekends, and you may have to find overflow parking along the road.

Take the Gabrielino Trail, which initially descends from the entrance to Chantry Flat into Big Santa Anita Canyon along a paved service road. Cross the Winter Creek Bridge at 0.6 mile and walk up the broad canyon trail, passing numerous private cabins, to a four-way trail junction at 1.4 miles. Continue straight ahead. You ford Big Santa Anita Creek in 200 yards, and then reford where the canyon makes a sharp bend left. Scramble over boulders the last 100 yards to the large pool at the foot of the falls (GPS N34° 12.704' W118° 01.168'). *Caution:* People have been injured trying to climb the falls.

Return the way you came. The hardest part is the final heartbreak hill back to the trailhead.

■ Hike 37 MOUNT ZION LOOP ○ 🐎 🥾

HIKE LENGTH 8.5-mile loop; 2,000' elevation gain
DIFFICULTY Moderate
SEASON November–June
MAP Tom Harrison *Angeles Front Country*
PERMIT Post Adventure Pass, or park on road outside fee area.

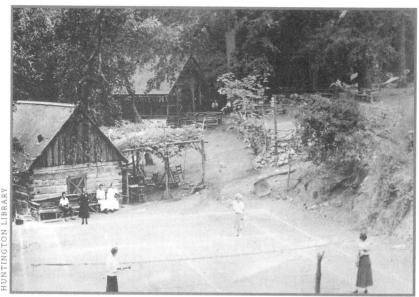

Sturtevant Camp in the early days

■ FEATURES

Note: This hike is within the Bobcat Fire Closure Area and is closed at least through April 1, 2022. Parts of Big Santa Anita Canyon burned severely. Check with the U.S. Forest Service (fs.usda.gov/angeles) before visiting.

This attractive loop hike follows the old Sturtevant Trail, known today as the Upper Winter Creek Trail, from Chantry Flat to Hoegees Trail Camp, and climbs over Mount Zion Saddle and drops into upper Big Santa Anita Canyon. You then follow the canyon trail down past Sturtevant Camp, Spruce Grove Trail Camp, and Cascade Picnic Area to lower Winter Creek and then climb back up to Chantry Flat. This is a delightful circle trip—one of the best in the San Gabriels—passing across chaparral-coated slopes with expansive canyon views, through lush conifer forest and streamside woodland, and alongside bubbling creeks, fully sampling the grandeur of the Big Santa Anita watershed.

Big Santa Anita Canyon is, perhaps, the most beautiful wooded glen in the San Gabriels, a favorite sylvan retreat for nature lovers, hikers, and campers. Under spreading evergreens, the musical waters of Big Santa Anita Creek reveal a delightful diversity of moods—now dancing merrily over a pebble-strewn floor, then pausing in a limpid pool, only to plunge headlong over a waterfall and cascade to begin a new cycle. Along the banks sprout regal Woodwardia ferns, dotted here and there in springtime with clusters of lupines, larkspurs, and other flowering herbs, all contributing to nature's soft picture of elegance.

The canyon has a rich history. In the 1850s there was a gold strike in the lower canyon, just about where Santa Anita Dam and Reservoir are now. The excitement lasted a few years, and then the miners drifted away. In 1886–1887, the Burlingame brothers constructed a rough road along the west slopes of the canyon to Winter Creek, intent on hauling out timber to fire their charcoal kilns. But the San Gabriels were declared a timber reserve before the brothers could cut any trees.

Wilbur Sturtevant, known as Sturde to his friends, built his trail from Sierra Madre over the ridge into Big Santa Anita Canyon, and then along the west slope to his resort camp in 1896. For decades, the famous Sturtevant Trail felt the trod of many boots and heard the joyous voices of legions of hikers bound for the delights of Big Santa Anita and its many hostelries of the Great Hiking Era. One who hiked the Sturtevant Trail and fell in love with alder-and-fern-lined Winter Creek was Arie Hoegee, who built his resort camp there in 1908. For three decades it was a favorite destination for hikers. The rustic buildings are long gone, but the U.S. Forest Service has made the little streamside glen into Hoegees Trail Camp, with stoves and tables. Hoegees Trail Camp has an unusual distinction: in the 24-hour period of January 22–23, 1942, a total of 26.12 inches of rain fell here, establishing a Southern California record that still stands.

Detracting somewhat from the primeval scene are the dozens of check dams, built of precast concrete and interlocked like giant Lincoln logs, which have converted the once-rustic canyon bottom into a progression of artificial stairsteps, with glassy sheets of water pouring over 10- to 20-foot drops. These check dams were constructed by the Los Angeles County Flood Control District and the Forest Service in the early 1960s as safeguards against erosion, much to the disgust of conservationists. Fortunately, 40 years of nature's regrowth have softened the appearance of artificiality, and the canyon has regained much of its former beauty.

This circle trip was made possible by the restoration of the Mount Zion section of the Sturtevant Trail by Howard Casebolt, Chris Kasten, and

Bohdan Porendowski of Camp Sturtevant from 1976 to 1979, and The Big Santa Anita Gang and Sierra Club volunteers from 1984 to 1985.

Bears are a constant nuisance in this canyon, especially at Hoegees Camp. If you camp here, be sure to bring a bear canister to store your food; hanging your food is not reliable and encourages bears to continue harassing campers in the hopes of finding food.

■ DESCRIPTION

From the 210 Freeway in Arcadia, take Exit 32 for Santa Anita Avenue. Drive north 5 miles to the parking lots at Chantry Flat (GPS N34° 11.734' W118° 01.347'), passing a gate open 6 a.m.–8 p.m. The popular trailhead fills early on weekends, and you may have to find overflow parking along the road.

From the upper parking area, hike 0.25 mile up a fire road. At the road's second switchback, turn right onto the Upper Winter Creek Trail, indicated by a wooden sign. Follow the trail as it climbs, contours, and then drops along the west wall of Big Santa Anita Canyon, mostly through chaparral, passing a Mount Wilson Trail junction to Winter Creek in 2.4 miles. Your trail fords Winter Creek, briefly climbs, and then drops to the Mount Zion/ Hoegees Trail Camp trail junction at 2.5 miles. For Hoegees Trail Camp, go right; the trail passes the Mount Zion Trail junction, refords Winter Creek, and reaches the tree-shaded camp after a few minutes' walk. (An option that cuts your hiking distance in half is to descend the Lower Winter Creek Trail to the Gabrielino Trail, then turn right and climb back up to Chantry Flat.)

To complete the full loop, retrace your steps from Hoegees Trail Camp back up to the signed Mount Zion Trail junction. Go right and follow the restored Mount Zion Trail (which is really the upper section of the old Sturtevant Trail) as it climbs, first through forest and then through chaparral, to Zion Saddle at 4.0 miles. A side trail to the right leads 0.1 mile to Mount Zion's summit and spectacular views over the Big Santa Anita watershed. Your main trail then gently descends through lush forest, mostly big-cone Douglas-firs, to Sturtevant Camp at 4.9 miles. You may rent cabins here with advance reservations; see sturtevantcamp.com.

Turn right, then shortly right again to descend the Gabrielino Trail, fording the creek twice, to Spruce Grove Trail Camp at 5.2 miles. Continue down past Cascade Picnic Area at 5.7 miles. At Fallen Sign Junction, 6.2 miles, your trail splits and you may choose to take the easier upper horse trail or the lower and more scenic but rough and airy hiker trail; the two rejoin at 7.0 miles. Continue down past check dams and private canyons to the junction with Winter Creek at 7.8 miles, and then climb back up the paved road to Chantry Flat.

VARIATION   You can shorten this hike to 5 miles and 1,000 feet of elevation gain by making it an out-and-back to Hoegees Camp. Or start the hike in reverse for an out-and-back to Spruce Grove Trail Camp for a 6.5-mile trip with 1,600 feet of elevation gain. Both are popular overnight trips, especially for youth groups.

■ Hike 38 MOUNT WILSON VIA WINTER CREEK ↗ 🐕

HIKE LENGTH 6 miles one-way; 3,600' elevation gain
DIFFICULTY Strenuous (uphill)
SEASON November–June
MAP Tom Harrison *Angeles Front Country*
PERMIT Post Adventure Pass at Chantry Flat, or park on road outside fee area.

■ FEATURES

Note: This hike is within the Bobcat Fire Closure Area and is closed at least through April 1, 2022 Parts of Big Santa Anita Canyon burned severely. Check with the U.S. Forest Service (fs.usda.gov/angeles) before visiting.

Mount Wilson can be climbed by trails from more directions than any other peak in Southern California. This trip goes from Chantry Flat over the old Sturtevant Trail to Winter Creek, and then climbs steeply up through a dense forest of big-cone Douglas-firs and oaks to the Winter Creek–Little Santa Anita divide, where it joins the Old Mount Wilson Trail and continues to the toll road and the summit. A number of interesting variations can be planned (see below). Be in top physical shape; the trip is steeply uphill most of the way.

■ DESCRIPTION

This trip requires a 1-hour car shuttle (or ride-hailing service). For an uphill trip, leave your get-away vehicle at the Skyline Park Trailhead at the top of the Mount Wilson Trail. From the 210 Freeway in La Cañada Flintridge, drive 14 miles north and east on Highway 2 to Red Box Station and the

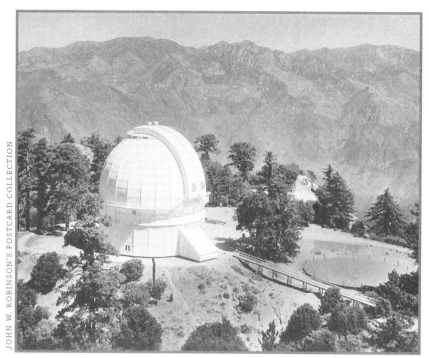

Mount Wilson Observatory

intersection of Mount Wilson Road at mile marker 2 LA 38.38. Turn right on Mount Wilson Road and proceed 4 miles to the parking lot at the end of the road (GPS N34° 13.379' W118° 03.772'). To reach the start of the hike, return to the 210 Freeway, drive east 11 miles, and take Exit 32 for Santa Anita Avenue. Drive north 5 miles to the parking lots at Chantry Flat (GPS N34° 11.734' W118° 01.347'), passing a vehicle gate open 6 a.m.–8 p.m. The trailhead fills early on weekends, and you may have to find overflow parking along the road.

From the upper parking area, hike 0.25 mile up a fire road. At the road's second switchback, turn right (northwest) onto the Sturtevant Trail (marked UPPER WINTER CREEK TRAIL on the topo map), and follow it around the ridges to a junction with the Mount Zion trail on the right at 2.4 miles. Stay left on the Winter Creek Trail, and continue climbing steeply through big-cone Douglas-firs and canyon live oaks to the ridgetop, where you join the Old Mount Wilson Trail coming up from Little Santa Anita Canyon at 4.5

miles (see Hike 35). Continue up the ridgetop trail as it zigzags steeply up, back and forth across the firebreak, to the Mount Wilson Toll Road at 5.1 miles. Turn right and follow the old toll road to the Harvard–Wilson saddle at 5.7 miles, then pick up a shortcut trail leading directly to the parking area at Skyline Park (6.2 miles).

VARIATIONS If you don't want to arrange a long car shuttle, you have many other options. You could return the way you came. You can enter Skyline Park (open April 1–November 30, with refreshments available Friday–Sunday, 10 a.m.–5 p.m.), walk past the observatory grounds to the east end of the mountain, and descend via the Sturtevant Trail (see Hike 39). Or, with a shorter car shuttle or ride-hailing service, you could follow the Mount Wilson Toll Road to Altadena (Hike 23) or the Old Mount Wilson Trail to Sierra Madre (Hike 35). Each of these options adds 7–8 miles, nearly all downhill.

You could also make this trip much easier by going one-way downhill.

■ Hike 39 MOUNT WILSON VIA STURTEVANT CAMP 🡕 🐐 🚶

HIKE LENGTH 7 miles one-way; 3,900' elevation gain
DIFFICULTY Strenuous (uphill)
SEASON November–June
MAP Tom Harrison *Angeles Front Country*
PERMIT Post Adventure Pass at Chantry Flat, or park on road outside fee area.

■ FEATURES

Note: This hike is within the Bobcat Fire Closure Area and is closed at least through April 1, 2022. Parts of Big Santa Anita Canyon burned severely. Check with the U.S. Forest Service (fs.usda.gov/angeles) before visiting.

The canyon of Big Santa Anita cuts a deep semicircular groove into the south flank of the front range, its head lying close under the precipitous east slope of Mount Wilson. An old trail travels most of the length of the canyon, then switchbacks steeply up forest- and chaparral-covered slopes to the mountaintop. This trip follows this old route, traveling upcanyon from Chantry Flat to Sturtevant Camp, then climbing right up the mountainside to Echo Rock and the observatory grounds. It is long and steep, so be in top shape.

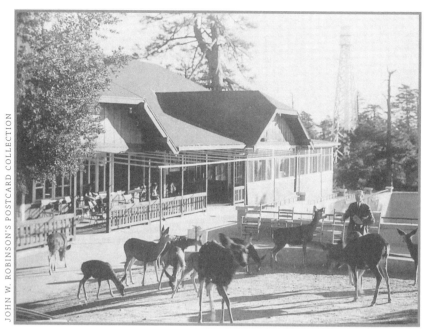

Mount Wilson Hotel (circa 1930)

■ DESCRIPTION

This trip requires a 1-hour car shuttle (or ride-hailing service). For an uphill trip, leave your getaway vehicle at the Skyline Park Trailhead at the top of the Mount Wilson Trail: From the 210 Freeway in La Cañada Flintridge, take the Angeles Crest Highway (Highway 2; Exit 20) 14 miles north and east to Red Box Station and the intersection of Mount Wilson Road at mile marker 2 LA 38.38. Turn right on Mount Wilson Road and proceed 4 miles to the parking lot at the end of the road (GPS N34° 13.379' W118° 03.772'). To reach the start of the hike, return to the 210 Freeway and drive east 11 miles. Take Exit 32 for Santa Anita Avenue and drive north 5 miles to the parking lots at Chantry Flat (GPS N34° 11.734' W118° 01.347'), passing a vehicle gate open 6 a.m.–8 p.m. The popular trailhead fills early on weekends, and you may have to find overflow parking along the road.

To the right of the road as you enter Chantry Flat, you will notice a locked gate and a paved fire road descending into the canyon. A large sign proclaims this road THE GABRIELINO RECREATION TRAIL (see Hike 40) and gives trail mileages. Follow this fire road to the canyon bottom at 0.6 mile,

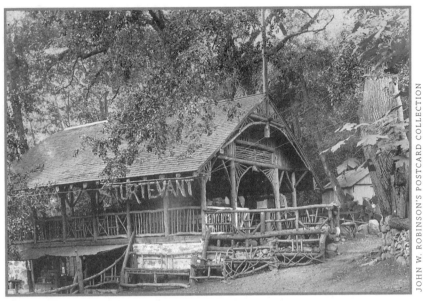

Sturtevant Camp

cross the Winter Creek Bridge, and walk up Big Santa Anita Canyon on the broad trail, passing numerous check dams and private cabins. At 1.3 miles you enter a shady recess and pass a cluster of cabins, once the site of Fern Lodge. Just beyond, the trail forks three ways: straight ahead to Sturtevant Falls (see Hike 36), left and then sharp right up the slope to climb above the falls into the middle canyon, and sharp left up the hillside to the upper canyon. Take either of the last two trails; they rejoin in a mile. The leftmost horse trail is easier walking, while the airier and more beautiful middle hiker trail leads directly above the falls and through the canyon. At 2.9 miles you drop back beside the alder- and bay-shaded stream and reach Cascade Picnic Area, on a forested bench to the right of the creek. Continue up the trail as it climbs the east slope and then drops to ford the creek and ascends to Spruce Grove Trail Camp at 3.5 miles. Youth groups frequent this campsite, which has stoves and tables.

Your trail climbs above the camp, fords the stream, and reaches a junction, the right fork going up to Newcomb Pass and on into the West Fork country (see Hike 44). This trip goes left; almost immediately, you reach the woodsy haunt of Sturtevant Camp, operating here since 1893 (4.0 miles; GPS N34° 13.325' W118° 02.114'). For years, the camp was operated as a

Methodist Church retreat, but since 2015, the cabins are open to the public with advance reservations (see sturtevantcamp.com).

Just before entering the camp, your trail turns sharply left and crosses the creek just above a debris barrier. Stay right on the Sturtevant Trail toward Mount Wilson, not left on the Mount Zion Trail. You now leave the canyon and switchback steeply up through dense big-cone Douglas-fir cover, which thins as you get higher, to Echo Rock at the east end of the Mount Wilson summit plateau, 6.6 miles from Chantry Flat. Walk through the observatory grounds to Skyline Park where your car awaits at 7.1 miles.

VARIATIONS If you don't want to set up a car shuttle, see the variations of Hike 38 for several descent options. Alternatively, you could make this trip much easier by going one-way downhill.

■ Hike 40 GABRIELINO NATIONAL RECREATION TRAIL ↗ 🐐 🚶

HIKE LENGTH 28 miles one-way; 4,800' elevation gain
DIFFICULTY Strenuous (2 days); moderate (3–4 days)
SEASON November–June
MAP Tom Harrison *Angeles Front Country*
PERMIT Post Adventure Pass at Chantry Flat, or park on road outside fee area.

■ FEATURES

Note: Parts of this hike are within the Bobcat Fire Closure Area and are closed at least through April 1, 2022. Segments between Chantry Flat and Red Box burned severely. Check with the U.S. Forest Service (fs.usda.gov/angeles) before visiting.

The Gabrielino National Recreation Trail was established by the Forest Service in 1970 as an outgrowth of the National Trails System Act passed by Congress. "This trail has been created for you—the city dweller—so that you might exchange, for a short time, the hectic scene of your urban life for the rugged beauty and freedom of adventure into the solitary wonderland of nature," read a Forest Service bulletin announcing the new trail.

Actually the trail is not new; it is a joining together and reworking of several old footpaths to form a semicircle over and around the central part of the front range. The name commemorates the Gabrielino Indians, who roamed these mountains long before the arrival of the white settlers in Southern

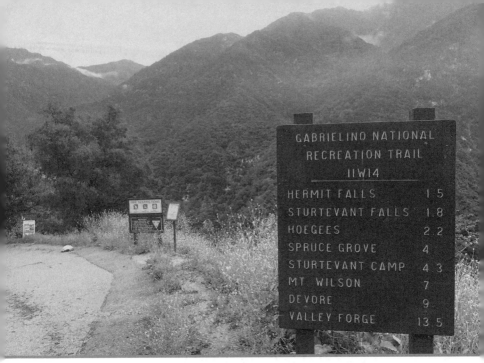

Southeastern terminus of the Gabrielino Trail at Chantry Flat

California, walking into the mountain canyons of the San Gabriels every summer to gather acorns and hunt wild game. In 1896 Will Sturtevant completed his trail into his resort camp at the head of Big Santa Anita Canyon. Louie Newcomb, another mountain pioneer who had settled in Chilao around 1888, decided that "Sturde's" footpath would make an excellent first leg for trips into his beloved backcountry. So with the help of 10 laborers, Newcomb thrashed out a rough pathway over the divide that now bears his name—Newcomb Pass—and down into the West Fork. Sturtevant and Newcomb attempted to charge a 25-cent toll for using their trail, but collecting was too difficult. The portion of the Gabrielino Trail up Arroyo Seco to Switzer's Camp also has a colorful history described in Hike 12.

The route covered in this trip starts at Chantry Flat and goes up Big Santa Anita Canyon, over Newcomb Pass, and down to the West Fork San Gabriel River along Newcomb's old route. It climbs to Red Box, descends Arroyo Seco, and finishes at Altadena. En route you sample the varied terrain and vegetation found in the front range: oak-shaded canyons, fir- and pine-dotted mountainsides, and chaparral-coated lower slopes.

This trip is best done as a three- or four-day backpack trip. You can camp overnight at any of six U.S. Forest Service campgrounds on the circular route. If you're in a monumental hurry, you can do it in two long days or even a single epic day.

■ **DESCRIPTION**

This hike begins at Chantry Flat and ends at Arroyo Seco, requiring a 16-mile car shuttle (or ride-hailing service). To leave your getaway vehicle at Arroyo Seco, take Exit 22B from the 210 Freeway for Windsor Avenue between Pasadena and La Cañada Flintridge. Go north 0.8 mile to the parking area at the corner of Ventura Street (GPS N34° 11.665' W118° 10.077'). To reach the starting point at Chantry Flat, return to the 210 and go east 9.3 miles to Exit 32 for Santa Anita Avenue. Drive north 5 miles to the parking lots at Chantry Flat (GPS N34° 11.734' W118° 01.347'), passing a vehicle gate open 6 a.m.–8 p.m. The lot fills early on weekends, so you may have to backtrack and park along the shoulder of the road.

The itinerary below is for a three-day outing. You can vary the trip to suit your own hiking pace and inclination.

DAY 1: Hike from Chantry Flat up the Big Santa Anita Canyon Trail, passing the first trail camp at Spruce Grove at 3.3 miles (GPS N34° 13.246' W118° 01.829'), and continue over Newcomb Pass (5.6 miles) and down to Devore Trail Camp on the West Fork San Gabriel River (7.1 miles; GPS N34° 14.597' W118° 02.149'). Spend your first night here, or continue to the West Fork Trail Camp at 8.2 miles (GPS N34° 14.772' W118° 02.981'). The trail fords the West Fork 10 times over this mile, and you are likely to get wet feet in the spring. If you get a late start from Chantry Flat, you can stay the night at Spruce Grove Trail Camp, adding an extra half day to the trip.

DAY 2: Hike up the West Fork, passing the Valley Forge campground off a spur (11.1 miles; GPS N34° 15.185' W118° 04.466'). Along the way, you will see the unmistakable effects of the 2009 Station Fire, which drastically altered the character of this once-lush portion of the trail. Cross the paved road at the Red Box parking area (13.2 miles; GPS N34° 15.481' W118° 06.287'), drop into the head of Arroyo Seco, and descend to Commodore Switzer Picnic Area at 17.4 miles (GPS N34° 15.969 W118° 08.718'). Continue down the wooded canyon to the former site of Commodore Switzer Trail Camp at 18.4 miles. There is no camping here, but if you need a place to spend the night, continue down to the junction with the Bear

Canyon Trail at 18.7 miles, and follow it down 0.4 mile to a junction with the Switzer Falls Trail on the left. Stay right and look for a legal campsite in a clearing off the right side of the trail shortly beyond (GPS N34° 15.285' W118° 09.069').

DAY 3: Back at the Bear Canyon Trail junction, continue down the Gabrielino Trail through the Arroyo Seco Trail (see Hike 12). The canyon widens near the Ken Burton Trail junction (22.2 miles). Pass the old site of Oakwilde Campground; little remains after the Station Fire. At 23.0 miles, the trail climbs onto the east wall of the canyon to bypass the Brown Canyon Debris Dam. Pass the Paul Little Picnic Area at 23.5 miles and the Nino Picnic Area at 24.5 miles before reaching Gould Mesa Campground at 25.0 miles (GPS N34° 13.342' W118° 10.704'). The remainder of the trip is easygoing, reaching the Windsor Avenue trailhead at 27.4 miles.

If you desire to do the trip in two days, the best overnight camp is Valley Forge Campground, midway up the West Fork. This will give you 11 miles of hiking the first day and a long, mostly downhill 17 miles on the second. Remember, you must camp in one of the authorized campgrounds.

■ Hike 41 MONROVIA CANYON FALLS 🡕 🐕 🚶

> **HIKE LENGTH** 2.6 miles out-and-back; 600' elevation gain
> **DIFFICULTY** Easy
> **SEASON** All year
> **MAP** Tom Harrison *Angeles High Country*
> **PERMIT** Pay $5 parking fee, or park on Canyon Boulevard.

■ FEATURES

Note: This hike was impacted by the 2020 Bobcat Fire and is temporarily closed. Check cityofmonrovia.org for the status of Monrovia Canyon Park.

Tucked away obscurely in two shady canyons behind the foothill community of Monrovia is one of the most beautiful parks in the Los Angeles area: Monrovia Canyon Park. Adding spice to the rich profusion of riparian vegetation is 40-foot-high Monrovia Canyon Falls, which runs with frothy exuberance for weeks or months after the rainy season ends.

The park is extremely popular, especially on pleasant weekends, so unless you arrive very early or on a weekday, you can expect to park on Canyon

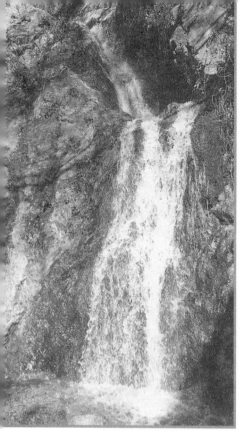

Monrovia Canyon Falls

Boulevard and walk 0.6 mile up the pavement to the trailhead.

Monrovia Canyon Park is open weekdays, 6:30 a.m.–6 p.m. The park is closed to vehicles on Tuesdays, but hikers are still permitted. The parking lot is also closed 5 p.m.–8 a.m. weekdays (until 7 a.m. weekends), so don't let your vehicle get locked inside.

Monrovia Canyon was homesteaded in 1874 by the Rankins family from Wisconsin. They made their living by selling wood that they cut at Sawpit Canyon, as well as by farming and beekeeping. The four children walked all the way to and from school in Duarte each day, until the eldest son died of typhoid fever at age 19; his two teenage sisters contracted it, too, and died a month later.

■ DESCRIPTION

From the 210 Freeway in Monrovia, take Exit 34 for Myrtle Avenue. Drive north 1.9 miles to where Myrtle Avenue ends at Scenic Drive. Turn right and follow Scenic Drive on a meandering eastward course for three blocks; then keep straight as Canyon Boulevard joins from the right. Proceed uphill on Canyon Boulevard, which crookedly ascends alongside the Sawpit Canyon wash to the park entrance. On most pleasant weekends, the small parking lots are overflowing by midmorning, and you'll have to park on Canyon Boulevard well short of the park entrance. Otherwise, pay an entrance fee and park in the small lot near the fee kiosk and ranger station (GPS N34° 10.369' W117° 59.487').

The signed Bill Cull Trail begins just above the fee kiosk. A fork on the right parallels and soon joins the road (optional return), but this trip stays left on the Bill Cull Trail, which was named for a dedicated volunteer trail builder. Switchbacks lead up to a junction at 0.2 mile with the Cunningham Overlook Trail on the left. Stay on the gorgeous main trail, which crosses Monrovia Creek at 0.6 mile, to a T-junction. Here, a nature trail leads right to the road, but you stay left. In another 0.1 mile, a second unsigned spur trail on the right leads to the nature center parking lot, but stay left again.

Your trail mostly sticks close to the canyon's sparkling stream, passing several check dams. Alder, oak, and bay trees cluster in the canyon bottom so densely that hardly any sunlight is admitted, even at midday. At 1.3 miles, the sound of splashing water heralds your arrival at the falls, where the stream either leaps or dribbles down two distinct declivities on a water-worn cliff face (GPS N34° 11.163' W117° 59.264').

Return the way you came, or take one of the spurs back to the park road and walk down the road, which is slightly shorter.

VARIATION The Cunningham Overlook Trail leads to a hill with good views of the valley below, adding 300 feet of climbing and 0.8 mile round-trip. The trail is named for Ed Cunningham, another volunteer trail builder who restored the path.

VARIATION If the parking lots are not full, you can drive all the way to the nature center parking area, shortening your hike to 1.6 miles round-trip but missing out on the scenic lower section.

■ Hike 42 BEN OVERTURFF TRAIL ◯ 🐕 ⚙

HIKE LENGTH 7-mile loop; 1,700' elevation gain
DIFFICULTY Moderate
SEASON All year
MAP Tom Harrison *Angeles High Country*
PERMIT Pay $5 parking fee, or park on Canyon Boulevard.

■ FEATURES

Note: This hike was impacted by the 2020 Bobcat Fire and is temporarily closed. Check cityofmonrovia.org for the status of Monrovia Canyon Park.

Beautiful Sawpit Canyon drains the southern slopes of Monrovia Peak. A lush canopy of alders and bays lines the creek. The slopes are blanketed with a thick cover of chaparral and, in the shadier recesses, oaks and big-cone

Douglas-firs. The city lies just over the ridge to the south, but here, you're in another world.

This pleasant trip begins at the lower end of Monrovia Canyon Park, follows the fire road up around Sawpit Canyon Reservoir, and then ascends the Overturff Trail to a little oak-shaded flat tucked into the south ramparts of Monrovia Peak known as Deer Park. The shady recess was discovered by Monrovia building contractor Ben Overturff around 1905. He built a stone cabin there, and for many years, from 1911 until the 1938 flood, Deer Park Lodge was a popular trail resort. Only the foundations remain today, under a canopy of majestic canyon oaks with a delightful all-year stream nearby.

Monrovia Canyon Park hours are Monday–Friday, 6:30 a.m.–6 p.m. The trail is sometimes closed Tuesdays or Wednesdays, when the Monrovia Police Department uses its Sawpit Canyon Shooting Range. Call the Monrovia Canyon Nature Center at 626-256-8282 for current information. The park is also closed to vehicles on Tuesdays but is still open to walk-in use.

■ DESCRIPTION

From the 210 Freeway in Monrovia, take Exit 34 for Myrtle Avenue. Drive north 1.9 miles to where Myrtle Avenue ends at Scenic Drive. Turn right and follow Scenic Drive on a meandering eastward course for three blocks, then keep straight as Canyon Boulevard joins from the right. Proceed uphill on Canyon Boulevard, which crookedly ascends alongside the Sawpit Canyon wash about a mile to the park entrance. On most pleasant weekends, the small parking lots are overflowing by midmorning and you will have to park on Canyon Boulevard well short of the park entrance. If the parking lot is open, pay the fee and park in the small lot near the fee kiosk and ranger station (GPS N34° 10.369' W117° 59.487').

Walk up the paved road briefly, then turn right onto Sawpit Fire Road, passing Sawpit Dam, built by the Los Angeles County Flood Control District in 1929, and, farther up, Trask Boy Scout Camp, both to your left. The road becomes unpaved just past the dam. At 1.3 miles, the road curves left and you reach the lower end of the Overturff Trail on your left, marked by a sign and two low stone pillars.

Follow the trail as it descends to Sawpit Creek, crosses it, and climbs to the Razorback, a sharp divide separating Sycamore and Sawpit Canyons. You follow the crest of the Razorback a short distance, and then climb the chaparral-covered slope to The Gap, a break in the ridge. Beyond, your pathway descends, contours, and gently climbs beneath a shady canopy of oaks and bay laurels. You reach Twin Springs Creek, where flowing water from one of the springs has formed a natural bridge. Just across the creek you pass a junction with a lateral trail that drops down to Sawpit Canyon fire road. You take the main trail straight ahead, climb over a low ridge, cross Deer Park Creek, and reach a second junction. Go left and climb 100 yards to Deer Park at 3.4 miles (GPS N34° 11.644' W117° 57.937'). Only the foundations remain of the once-popular lodge, shaded by tall oaks. It's a good picnic spot. Return the way you came, or drop down either of the two short lateral trails to Sawpit Fire Road, and follow the road back to your car.

■ Hike 43 FISH CANYON FALLS 🥾 🐕 🚶

> **HIKE LENGTH** 3.4 miles out-and-back; 600' elevation gain
> **DIFFICULTY** Easy
> **SEASON** Winter–summer, subject to access
> **MAP** Tom Harrison *Angeles High Country* (trail not shown)
> **PERMIT** N/A

■ FEATURES

Fish Canyon Falls are some of the top natural attractions of the San Gabriel Mountains. In spring, when the water runs high, the falls are a spectacular delight, plunging some 80 feet in stairway fashion. The topmost fall is the longest, shooting out from the narrow gorge above and then swishing down into a sparkling pool 40 feet below. Then there is a short cascade, followed by a 30-foot plunge into a lower pool, with one final 8-foot drop below that. A fine silver spray dampens the canyon walls when the water runs high, causing the walls to be embossed with lush green mosses and grasses. In the amphitheater below, aroar with the boom of the falls, there is a small flat, shaded by oaks and overhanging rock—a favorite spot for picnickers.

For decades, the canyon entrance was blocked by the quarrying operation of the Vulcan Materials Company. Various access methods included a horrible trail over Van Tassel Ridge and a seasonal shuttle through Vulcan's property. After years of litigation, the city and Vulcan Materials finally reached an agreement in 2014 and built a fenced trail through the quarry to reach the forest boundary. Shortly thereafter, the area was swept by the June

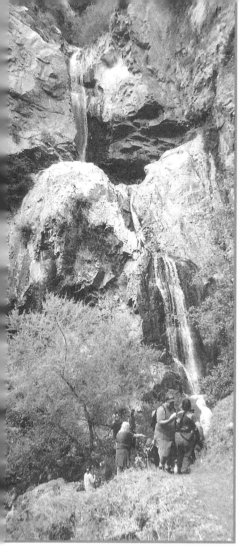

Hikers at Fish Canyon Falls
JOHN W. ROBINSON

2016 San Gabriel Complex Fire, and the trail has been closed ever since. The Van Tassel Ridge bypass trail was obliterated in the fire as well. Neither Vulcan nor the city appear to be in a hurry to restore access. Check with the U.S. Forest Service (fs.usda.gov/angeles) to see if this trail has reopened before you try to visit.

■ DESCRIPTION

From the northernmost end of I-605 in Duarte, turn right (east) on Huntington Drive. Proceed 0.6 mile east to Encanto Parkway. Turn left and follow Encanto Parkway (and its extension, Fish Canyon Road) northeast 1.4 miles. Turn left into the dirt parking lot (3901 Fish Canyon Road), which is just short of the Vulcan Materials rock quarry entrance.

Once you leave the quarry behind, this becomes a delightful hike. Your trail contours along the west slope of Fish Canyon about 50 feet above the creek, shaded by a canopy of live oaks, big-leaf maples, and alders. You pass the foundations of several cabins and then switchback higher up the canyon slope before dropping to the creek. You cross a small tributary stream, and then the main creek, and ascend the east slope to a sharp bend in the canyon where the falls abruptly come into view. Carefully descend the rocky slope to a shaded amphitheater alongside a shallow pool, just beneath the falls (GPS N34° 10.898' W117° 55.526'). Do not attempt to climb the falls, even though the rocks to the left look inviting. People have been severely injured trying. Return the way you came.

■ Hike 44 KENYON DEVORE TRAIL TO WEST FORK TRAIL CAMP ⤴ 🐕 🏃

HIKE LENGTH 8 miles out-and-back; 2,800' elevation gain
DIFFICULTY Moderate
SEASON All year
MAP Tom Harrison *Angeles Front Country*
PERMIT N/A

■ FEATURES

Note: This hike is within the Bobcat Fire Closure Area and is closed at least through April 1, 2022. Parts of the West Fork San Gabriel River watershed burned severely. Check with the U.S. Forest Service (fs.usda.gov/angeles) before visiting.

Kenyon DeVore (1911–1995) spent his whole life in and around the San Gabriel Mountains. He grew up at his parents' trail resorts on the West Fork San Gabriel River, first at Camp West Fork and then at Valley Forge Lodge. As a child, he busied himself with camp chores. As a teenager, he worked at the Mount Wilson Hotel and led a pack train that supplied resorts, forest stations, and campers throughout the mountains. DeVore spent most of his adult life working for the Los Angeles County Flood Control District, most of the time in San Gabriel Canyon. After his retirement in 1971, he signed on as an Angeles National Forest volunteer, and later as a part-time paid employee. For 15 years he was a familiar sight at the Chantry Flat visitor information station, giving advice and imparting knowledge to hikers, backpackers, and picnickers. It was only fitting that the old Rattlesnake Trail, which DeVore traveled many times with his pack train, be renamed in his honor.

The Kenyon DeVore Trail descends Strayns Creek from Mount Wilson to the West Fork San Gabriel. Despite its tortuous and coiling route down the steep canyon, it is one of the best trips in the San Gabriels. Situated entirely on a north-facing slope (the other Mount Wilson trails approach from the south or east), the path runs through lush forest all the way— Jeffrey and sugar pines, incense cedars, big-cone Douglas-firs, and many stands of oaks. Even on a warm day, this well-shaded trip is enjoyable. You cross Strayns Creek several times; in spring and early summer, the trickling water is ice cold and refreshing (but filter it).

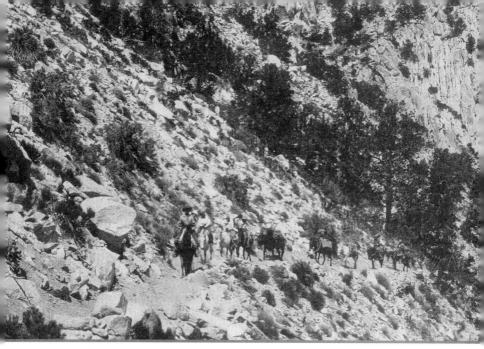

DeVore pack train on the Angeles Crest Trail   KENYON DEVORE

Strayns Canyon and Creek were named for A. G. Strain, who operated a resort camp near the upper head of the canyon from 1889 to 1917. The U.S. Geological Survey misspelled his name on the topo sheet, and the mistake has never been corrected.

This canyon is rich in history. Adjacent to West Fork Camp (not to be confused with Camp West Fork above), mountain pioneer Louie Newcomb hand-hewed a log cabin in 1900 that was the first ranger station in California and the second in the United States constructed with government funds ($70). Only the foundation remains today; the old ranger station was disassembled in 1982 and moved to Chilao, where it has been reassembled as a forestry museum behind the visitor center. Devore Trail Camp stands at the site of old Camp West Fork, a small wilderness resort set up by Ernest and Cherie DeVore in 1913. Camp West Fork was a favorite of anglers, most of whom made the trip in via the Sturtevant Trail from Sierra Madre over Newcomb Pass. It was also popular with hikers as a takeoff point for trips into the backcountry. The camp was abandoned after an ownership dispute in 1925, and now nothing remains of the old hostelry except the clearing now used as a U.S. Forest Service trail camp.

■ DESCRIPTION

Exit the 210 Freeway at Angeles Crest Highway (Highway 2; Exit 20) in La Cañada Flintridge. Drive 14 miles north and east to Red Box Station and the intersection of Mount Wilson Road at mile marker 2 LA 38.38. Turn right on Mount Wilson Road and proceed 4.4 miles to where the road splits and becomes a one-way loop around the antenna-spiked Mount Wilson ridgeline. Parking space is available in a roadside turnout to the west (GPS N34° 13.662' W118° 04.056').

The trail drops north through an oak forest along the west slope of Strayns Canyon. Switchback down through open stands of pines, cross the creek, and contour high along the east slope before switchbacking down to the creek and fording it again to the west slope. Then you descend through a shady pine forest, recross Strayns Creek, and drop to a junction with the Gabrielino Trail at 2.6 miles. Most of the trees in this section were burned away in 2009; you pass through the charred stumps of what used to be forest. Follow the trail east, along the south slope of the canyon, down to West Fork Trail Camp at 4.1 miles (GPS N34° 14.772 W118° 02.981'). Here, the fire damage is mostly confined to the slopes north of the stream; the campground remains a sylvan delight with stoves, tables, and toilets. It is reached by dirt road from Red Box, but as of this writing the road is closed to public traffic. Return the way you came.

VARIATIONS The West Fork San Gabriel River has three fine trail camps (Valley Forge, West Fork, and Devore), all of which receive far less use than the Chantry and Arroyo Seco areas nearby. Studying the map reveals many options for loop and out-and-back hikes, mostly involving substantial descents and climbs.

For example, hike down from Mount Wilson Road to the bottom of the DeVore Trail, turn west, and hike 1.5 miles to Valley Forge Trail Camp (0.2 mile down a spur off the Gabrielino Trail). Then return to the Valley Forge Trail, and follow it steeply back up to Eaton Saddle, a total of 7 miles with 2,100 feet of elevation gain. This option requires a 2.0-mile car, bike, or jogging shuttle along Mount Wilson Road to close the loop.

Another excellent option is to hike the DeVore Trail to West Fork Trail Camp, then continue along the Gabrielino Trail, repeatedly fording the river, to Devore Trail Camp and then up to Newcomb Pass. Turn onto the the Rim

Trail, and follow it up the unrelenting ridge to Mount Wilson. This loop is 11 miles with 2,500 feet of elevation gain.

From Red Box, you could hike the Gabrielino Trail 2.3 miles to Valley Forge Trail Camp, and then either retrace your steps or, with a shuttle, exit via the Valley Forge, Kenyon DeVore, Silver Moccasin, or Rim Trail or continue out to Chantry Flat.

▪ Hike 45 SHORTCUT CANYON TO WEST FORK TRAIL CAMP 🥾 🐕 🏃

LENGTH 7 miles out-and-back; 1,800' elevation gain
DIFFICULTY Moderate
SEASON November–May
MAP Tom Harrison *Angeles Front Country*
PERMIT Free first-come, first-served campground

▪ FEATURES

Note: This hike is within the Bobcat Fire Closure Area and is closed at least through April 1, 2022. Parts of the West Fork San Gabriel River watershed burned severely. Check with the U.S. Forest Service (fs.usda.gov/angeles) before visiting.

Years ago, before the Angeles Crest Highway was a reality, Shortcut Canyon felt the trod of many boots and hooves. Its busy trail, built in 1893 by Louie Newcomb, Arthur Carter, and John Hartwell, was the major route into the Charlton Flat–Chilao–Buckhorn backcountry. The canyon and trail were so named because they greatly cut the distance into the mountain interior. The old route, which has now completely disappeared, was the steep Native American footpath up Valley Forge Canyon and over Barley Flats. Newcomb thrashed out a rough pathway over the divide that now bears his name (Newcomb Pass), down into the West Fork, and then up Shortcut Canyon and on to his Chilao country. While Newcomb was working on his path, Sturtevant and several others incorporated the Sierra Madre and Antelope Valley Toll Trail and charged 25 cents per person to hike across the range to the desert, with the first fares going to Newcomb for his part in building the trail. However, Newcomb, who had to do the collecting himself, complained that no system of collection would work without someone on the trail at all times, and "that don't pay wages, so I had to quit it." Although the old Shortcut pathway is no longer a major artery of travel, it is part of the Boy Scouts' Silver Moccasin Trail across the range from Red Box to Mount Baden-Powell (see Hike 74).

Most of the trees burned in the 2009 Station Fire, but the chaparral has recovered. Along the stream, the West Fork still retains the charm of yesteryear. You will get the feel of the old San Gabriels, when bandits, hunters, anglers, and prospectors rambled into the then-wild heart of the range. Watch for blackberry brambles, which ripen in the summer. Most of this hike is now shadeless due to the fire, so do it on a cool day and bring plenty of water.

■ **DESCRIPTION**

Exit the 210 Freeway at Angeles Crest Highway (Highway 2; Exit 20) in La Cañada Flintridge. Drive 19 miles north and east to Shortcut Saddle at mile marker 2 LA 43.3 (GPS N34° 16.411' W118° 01.959').

From the saddle, take the Silver Moccasin/Shortcut Canyon Trail, which leads south. After several short switchbacks you reach a fire road; turn right (west) and follow the fire road about 200 yards, to where you again pick up the trail leading down to your left. You drop steeply down chaparral-covered slopes into the East Fork of Shortcut Canyon. Your path now descends the shady canyon floor, rough in places, and passes the junction of Shortcut's West Fork as you cross and recross the trickling creek. At 3.5 miles you reach the broad West Fork San Gabriel River. Boulder-hop across the creek (this could be dangerous in times of high water) and reach West Fork Trail Camp, located on a forested bench south of the river (GPS N34° 14.772' W118° 02.981'). The campground has stoves, tables, and toilets. The historic West Fork Ranger Station, built here in 1900 and the second-oldest in the nation, was moved to the Chilao Visitor Center in the early 1980s. Relax along the canopied creek before heading back up Shortcut Canyon to your car.

VARIATIONS You could continue to Devore Trail Camp, 1.1 miles and many stream crossings down the West Fork. With a car or bicycle shuttle you can ascend the Kenyon DeVore Trail to Mount Wilson (4.2 miles from West Fork Trail Camp; see Hike 44) or take the Gabrielino Trail (see Hike 40) 5.0 miles west to Red Box or 8.4 miles southeast to Chantry Flat.

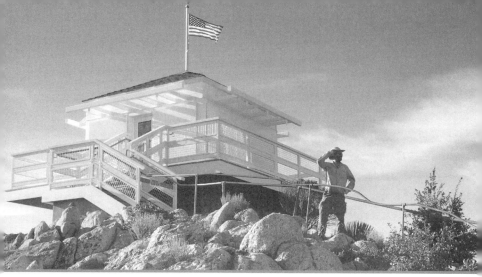

The newly rebuilt Vetter Mountain Fire Lookout escaped the 2020 Bobcat Fire.

■ Hike 46 VETTER MOUNTAIN ↻ 🐕 👫

HIKE LENGTH 3.6-mile loop; 700' elevation gain
DIFFICULTY Easy
SEASON All year
MAP Tom Harrison *Angeles Front Country*
PERMIT N/A

■ FEATURES

Note: This hike is within the Bobcat Fire Closure Area and is closed at least through April 1, 2022. Portions of this hike around Charlton Flats burned, but the new fire lookout escaped the fire. Check with the U.S. Forest Service (fs.usda.gov/angeles) before visiting.

The Vetter Mountain Fire Lookout is perched atop the 5,908-foot summit and offers a 360-degree view over the midsection of the San Gabriels. The lookout was rebuilt in 2019 after being destroyed in the 2009 Station Fire. This is a good place to fully appreciate the extent of the Station and Bobcat Fire burn areas across the western and central thirds of the mountain range. The mountain is named for Victor Vetter, a ranger and dispatcher active around 1930.

Aside from visiting Vetter's summit, this loop hike also swings around through Charlton Flats' formerly lush, heterogeneous forest of live oak, Coulter pine, ponderosa pine, incense cedar, and big-cone Douglas-fir. In the years to come it will be interesting to observe the pattern of plant succession, and to learn just how much of the forest has survived and which kinds of trees will be favored in the postfire environment.

■ DESCRIPTION

Exit the 210 Freeway at Angeles Crest Highway (Highway 2; Exit 20) in La Cañada Flintridge. Drive 23 miles north and east to the turnoff for Charlton Flats Picnic Area on the left at mile marker 2 LA 47.54. After turning into the picnic area, swing right at the first intersection and continue 0.6 mile to a gate. Park just short of the gate, observing signed parking restrictions (GPS N34° 17.889' W118° 00.873').

Take the signed trail to Vetter Mountain, starting up the south side of a ravine. About 200 yards up the path, the Silver Moccasin Trail swings left—don't take it; this is your return route. Keeping straight, you ascend through mixed forest and then scattered pines, crossing paved service roads twice. A final switchbacking stretch through chaparral leads to the lookout site, 1.3 miles from the start (GPS N34° 17.825' W118° 01.717').

Looking north and east from the lookout perch, you'll spot Pacifico Mountain, Mount Williamson, Waterman Mountain, Twin Peaks, Old Baldy, and other High Country summits. The Front Range sprawls west and south, blocking from view most of the city. Most of the Angeles National Forest west and north of Vetter was incinerated in the Station Fire, and chaparral has largely replaced the trees.

When it's time to descend, follow the dirt road downhill instead of the trail. At 2.0 miles you'll join a paved service road. Continue straight (east) on the pavement to reach the Silver Moccasin Trail at 2.6 miles. Turn left on the trail, cross pavement again, and complete the final, mostly level stretch across a forested slope.

■ Hike 47 PACIFICO MOUNTAIN 🏃 🐕 🥾

HIKE LENGTH 10 miles out-and-back; 1,700' elevation gain
DIFFICULTY Moderate
SEASON May–October
MAP Tom Harrison *Angeles Front Country* and *Angeles High Country*
PERMIT N/A

■ FEATURES

Pacifico Mountain looms high on the northern rampart of the San Gabriels, offering far-reaching panoramas over Antelope Valley and the Mojave Desert. On days when the sky is clear of the usual desert haze, the viewer can make out, on the distant horizon, the sawtooth peaks of the High Sierra and the distinct cone-shaped summit of Telescope Peak overlooking Death Valley.

Legend says that 7,124-foot Pacifico Mountain and its all-year spring were a hangout of Tiburcio Vásquez and his gang of horse thieves in the 1870s. In fact, the infamous bandido supposedly gave it the name Pacifico because he could see the Pacific Ocean from the top.

This pleasant, view-rich trip follows the easy-graded Pacific Crest Trail most of the way. Part of the area burned in the 2009 Station Fire, leaving a crazy quilt of new growth and pristine forest. Backpackers can spend the night free of charge at a small first-come, first-served campground on the boulder-studded summit, a perfect spot for watching the sunrise (but bring your own water).

You can drive to Mount Pacifico Campground from the west or east via dirt Forest Road 3N17. This could facilitate a one-way trip or a campout for a youth group. Check with the U.S. Forest Service (fs.usda.gov/angeles) before relying on the road because it sometimes washes out.

■ DESCRIPTION

From the 210 Freeway in La Cañada Flintridge, take the Angeles Crest Highway (Highway 2; Exit 20) north and east 28.2 miles to Sulphur Springs Road at mile marker 2 LA 52.85. Turn left onto Sulphur Springs Road and go 3.9 miles to a fork at Alder Saddle; then turn right on paved one-lane FR 5N04. In 1.0 mile, park at a clearing on the right, immediately beyond the turnoff for Sulphur Springs Campground.

From the parking area, walk back along the road 150 yards to find the signed Pacific Crest Trail (GPS N34° 22.264' W117° 59.919'). Follow it west-northwest as it winds above a drainage. The rather unimpressive, partially burned hill on the skyline is Pacifico Mountain. The PCT gradually climbs through scrub oak and mountain mahogany and the occasional Coulter pine. This area is notable for flannel bush, which lights up the trail with vivid yellow flowers in the spring.

Pass through a burn zone, and then round a bend onto the west side of a ridge, where you'll find shade under black oaks that escaped the inferno. At 2.5 miles, reach a prominent saddle. At 3.0 miles, pass seasonal Fiddleneck Spring, surrounded by ferns and shaded by an incense cedar.

At 3.6 miles, pass Fountainhead Spring, which is more robust but still not reliable after springtime.

At 4.3 miles, reach a flat on the pine-covered north ridge of Pacifico Mountain (GPS N34° 23.337' W118° 01.716'). Depart the PCT and make a cross-country ascent to the summit, weaving past the granite boulders on the ridge. Your climb ends abruptly at Pacifico Mountain Campground, where you'll find 10 tent sites shaded beneath the Jeffrey and sugar pines, white firs, and incense cedars. The true high point is a 20-foot boulder at 4.9 miles (GPS N34° 22.918' W118° 02.070'). The climb is tricky and a fall could have nasty consequences. Most hikers will be satisfied by taking a snack break at the base.

You can return the way you came or make a loop by returning on dirt roads. The road walk adds a mile but is fast, easy going. Follow the campground access road, FR 3N17H, 1.6 miles down to FR 3N17. Turn left and go 3.2 miles to Alder Saddle. Turn left again on FR 5N04 and follow it 1.0 mile back to your vehicle.

VARIATION Pacifico Mountain can also be climbed by way of the Pacific Crest Trail from Mill Creek Summit on the Angeles Forest Highway. This round-trip hike is 13 miles in length with 2,300 feet of elevation gain. Follow the PCT up to a saddle where the trail meets FR 3N17H. Turn left and follow the road 1.1 miles to the summit. Return to the junction, then follow FR 3N17H down to FR 3N17. Turn right and follow the road back to Mill Creek Summit.

■ Hike 48 DEVILS CANYON 🡕 🐕 🚶

HIKE LENGTH 6 miles out-and-back; 1,500' elevation loss and gain
DIFFICULTY Moderate
SEASON November–April
MAP Tom Harrison *Angeles Front Country* and *Angeles High Country*
PERMIT Post Adventure Pass, or park outside fee area.

■ FEATURES

Note: This hike is within the Bobcat Fire Closure Area and is closed at least through April 1, 2022. It appears that Devils Canyon did not burn. Check with the U.S. Forest Service (fs.usda.gov/angeles) before visiting.

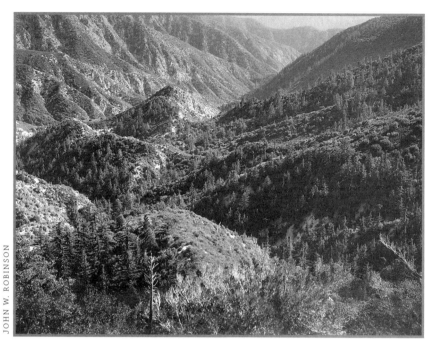

Devils Canyon, San Gabriel Wilderness

Fewer than 20 air miles from downtown Los Angeles is the San Gabriel Wilderness, 36,000 acres of rugged ridge and canyon country forever protected and preserved in its natural state. There are no roads, resorts, or noisy public campgrounds, only the primeval sounds of earth— the wind rustling the leaves of pines and alders; the stream dancing over boulders and cascades; the wren-tit's staccato call; and, on rare occasions, the mountain lion darting through brush. Only three maintained trails enter this wilderness. Perhaps the most delightful one leaves the Angeles Crest at Chilao and descends steep slopes of chaparral, firs, and pines into the shaded bowels of Devils Canyon. Here, under a green canopy of alders and willows, alongside deep pools and miniature waterfalls, the hiker can find solitude on a day's outing or overnight backpack, and relive a part of the mountains as they once were. Take care; this is an "upside-down" trip— downhill all the way in, uphill on the return. Many an out-of-condition rambler has stridden gaily down, only to labor painfully every upward step out. Avoid this trip on a hot day.

■ DESCRIPTION

Exit the 210 Freeway at Angeles Crest Highway (Highway 2; Exit 20) in La Cañada Flintridge. Drive 26 miles north and east to the Devils Canyon Trailhead on the right at mile marker 2 LA 50.50, just south of the Chilao Visitor Center turnoff (GPS N34° 19.423' W118° 00.175').

The trail, well maintained by the U.S. Forest Service, is easy to follow. It loses no time in descending the steep hillsides, alternately through stands of big-cone Douglas-firs on shady north faces and through dense chaparral on sunnier slopes. About halfway down, the trail meets a small tributary creek and then follows it to the main canyon. Continue a few hundred yards downstream to a wilderness camping area on a shaded bench on your right, well above the stream (2.8 miles; GPS N34° 18.595' W117° 58.986'). You might enjoy lunch or a night here before returning the way you came. Allow plenty of time for the return trip—at least twice what it took to get in. Remember, it's all uphill.

VARIATION It is possible, without inordinate difficulty for the average hiker, to follow Devils Canyon downstream about 2 miles—crossing and recrossing the creek, boulder-hopping, and occasionally thrashing through willow and brush. A 20-foot waterfall blocks further travel unless you are equipped with technical gear.

■ Hike 49 MOUNT HILLYER ◘ ⇥ 🕅 🕅

HIKE LENGTH 6-mile loop; 1,000' elevation gain
DIFFICULTY Moderate
SEASON All year
MAP Tom Harrison *Angeles Front Country*
PERMIT N/A

■ FEATURES

The Chilao–Horse Flats country is a gentle region of rounded ridgetops, shallow draws, and small flats set deep in the heart of the San Gabriels. The forest here is open and parklike; tall Jeffrey pines and incense cedars cluster in sheltered recesses and dot the rolling hillsides. The chaparral is rich and green, and the sky is a deep blue, with seldom a trace of the brown murkiness that so often invades the south slope of the range. This is ideal picnicking, camping, and hiking country.

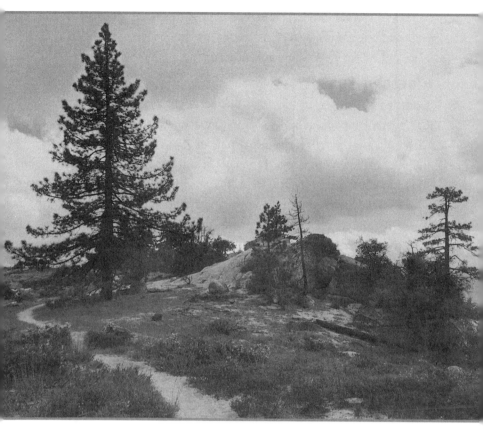

Jeffrey pines and granite boulders on the summit of Mount Hillyer

A century ago this was bandido country. The notorious Tiburcio Vásquez and his gang of horse thieves used Chilao and Horse Flats—at that time deep in the wilderness and little known—as refuges from the law, as hideouts where they could rest and plan their next raid, and as pastures for stolen horses. The great boulders of nearby Mount Hillyer furnished an impregnable fortress if pursuing posses came too close. One of Vásquez's men at Chilao was a herder named Jose Gonzales, noted among his cohorts for his skill with a knife. On one occasion he killed a bear with some slick knife work, earning the nickname Chillia ("hot stuff"). From this allegedly came the name Chilao.

There are no bandidos here now, and roads lace the region, but the country still holds appeal. This scenic trail hike takes you through the best of the Chilao–Horse Flats area, and it climbs through magnificent stands of Jeffrey pines and around jumbo granite boulders to the summit of Mount Hillyer. Rock climbers may enjoy trying their skill on the boulder problems near Horse Flats and Hillyer (search for Horse Flats on mountainproject.com).

■ DESCRIPTION

Exit the 210 Freeway at the Angeles Crest Highway (Highway 2; Exit 20) in La Cañada Flintridge. Drive 26 miles north and east to the turnoff for the Chilao Visitor Center on the left at mile marker 2 LA 50.60. Take this road 0.6 mile (passing the visitor center) to a small parking area for the Silver Moccasin Trail on the right (GPS N34° 19.866' W118° 00.722'). If the Chilao road is closed to vehicles in the winter, park at the turnoff and walk in.

Proceed 1.0 mile up the trail as it switchbacks through chaparral and clusters of Jeffrey pines—the 2009 Station Fire did some damage here—to a junction just short of Horse Flats Campground. Turn left, leaving the

The Mount Hillyer Trail meanders through Jeffrey pines and sagebrush reminiscent of the Sierra Nevada Mountains.

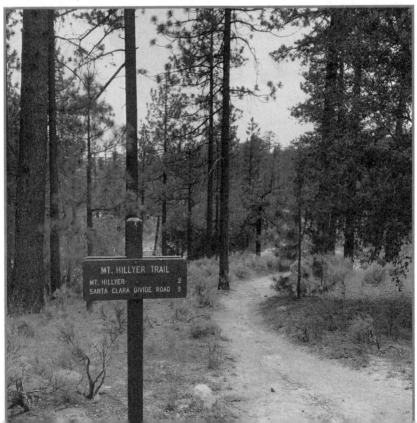

Silver Moccasin Trail, and follow the path 100 yards to the south edge of the campground (first-come, first served; no water). A sign to your left indicates MT. HILLYER, 2 MILES. Proceed up the Mount Hillyer Trail through open clusters of manzanitas, scrub oaks, and Jeffrey pines and around a maze of giant granite boulders, to the broad summit of Mount Hillyer at 2.4 miles (GPS N34° 20.792' W118° 01.254'). You can't see much from the forested top, but if you walk several hundred feet southwest onto the firebreak, you are rewarded with a fine panorama of the rolling bandido country to the south and southeast, and the broad trench of fire-scorched Alder Creek dropping off to the west.

You could return the same way, but to make a pleasant semiloop, go north from the summit along the ridgetop trail, which climbs gently over two nubbins before descending to a junction with the Santa Clara Divide Road (3N17) at 3.3 miles. Turn right (southeast) to follow the paved road, and then right again at 3.8 miles on the Horse Flats Campground access road to Horse Flats, where you meet your trail of ascent. From here, follow the same route down to your car.

VARIATION You can shorten this trip to 3.6 miles and 700 feet of elevation gain by driving to Horse Flats Campground (GPS N34° 20.451' W118° 00.596'). Turn left off Angeles Crest Highway at mile marker 2 LA 52.85, where a sign indicates SANTA CLARA DIVIDE ROAD, and proceed 2.5 miles on this road to the campground.

■ Hike 50 TWIN PEAKS AND MOUNT WATERMAN TRAVERSE ✎ 🐎 🚶

    HIKE LENGTH 13 miles one-way; 4,000' elevation gain
    DIFFICULTY Strenuous
    SEASON June–October
    MAP Tom Harrison *Angeles High Country*
    PERMIT Post Adventure Pass at Three Points, or park outside fee area.

■ FEATURES

Note: This hike is within the Bobcat Fire Closure Area and is closed at least through April 1, 2022. Patches of the forest on these mountains burned. Check with the U.S. Forest Service (fs.usda.gov/angeles) before visiting.

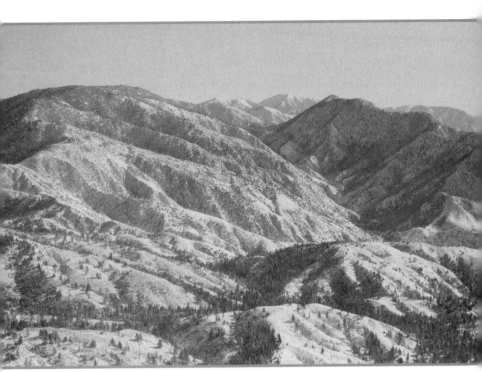

Aerial view of Waterman (left) and Twin Peaks (right) framing Mount Baldy (distant skyline)

This trip traverses the high country along the northern boundary of the San Gabriel Wilderness and climbs the two major peaks in the region. From the ramparts of Twin Peaks, you look down over the rugged upper reaches of Devils and Bear Canyons, the wildest mountain country in the San Gabriels. Here, among the crags and in the deep recesses, are the undisturbed lairs of mountain lions, black bears, and bighorn sheep, animals seldom seen in the more frequented parts of the range.

This is delightful wilderness country. The topography is more broken than in most other parts of the range, and jumbo boulders dot the slopes. The chaparral is tall and richly textured. The forest, primarily Jeffrey and ponderosa pines, is open and parklike, carpeted with pine needles. Near Twin Peaks Saddle are some of the most beautiful stands of incense cedars in the range. On sunny slopes, lupines stand bright and pagodalike in early summer. Half a dozen trickling rills line the route during early season, only to disappear one by one as the dry months progress.

A car shuttle between Three Points and Buckhorn is required if you wish to do the full traverse. Although the total trip is classified as strenuous, parts of it can be done and thoroughly enjoyed by the neophyte. A 2-mile stroll up-trail from Three Points will reward the beginner with superb vistas into Devils Canyon. If you are a hiker of moderate ability, you can continue 4 more miles to Twin Peaks Saddle and return. This high wilderness is too good to be reserved for only the strongest; it is there for all.

■ **DESCRIPTION**

This trip requires a 5-mile car or bicycle shuttle. Leave your getaway vehicle at the Buckhorn Trailhead. To get there, from the 210 Freeway in La Cañada Flintridge, take the Angeles Crest Highway (Highway 2; Exit 20) 33 miles north and east to the Buckhorn Trailhead at mile marker 2 LA 58.00 (GPS

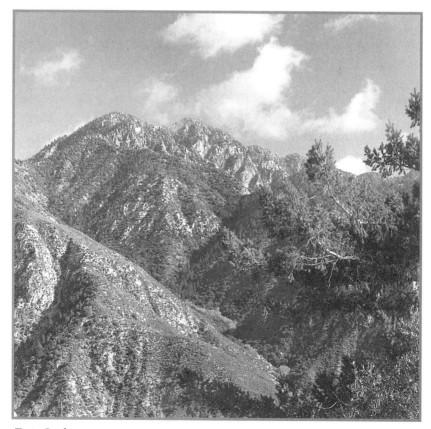

Twin Peaks   JOHN W. ROBINSON

N34° 20.819' W117° 55.294'). Then return 5.2 miles to the Three Points Trailhead at mile 52.8 by the intersection of Santa Clara Divide Road (GPS N34° 20.599' W117° 58.985').

From the parking area just above Three Points, take the trail that leads down to the Pacific Crest Trail (PCT) 50 yards. Turn left and follow the PCT down to the highway, which must be crossed with care (on weekends some vehicles and motorcycles use the Angeles Crest as a speedway). Pick up the PCT on the east side of the highway. The PCT begins climbing above the highway, and in about 100 yards you reach a junction. Here, you leave the PCT and go right for Mount Waterman. Your trail starts zigzagging up the west spine of the mountain. There is evidence of the 2009 Station Fire here—the eastern edge of the burn area. After gaining about 600 feet, the route levels off and traverses around the long, indented slopes of Waterman. The deep trench of Devils Canyon is constantly in view to your right. Keep a sharp lookout for bighorn sheep; they are occasionally seen here. The trail rounds the mountain and at 4.8 miles reaches a junction—left up to Mount Waterman, right down to Twin Peaks Saddle. Go right, descending 400 feet to Twin Peaks Saddle at 5.6 miles. You could find pleasant but dry dispersed camping here. The maintained trail ends here, but a pathway worn by climbers, steep in places, leads up the north slope of Twin Peaks 1,200 feet to the summit at 6.7 miles (GPS N34° 18.953' W117° 55.599'); the eastern of the two peaks is higher. This is the climax of the trip. From the top you see nature's pattern of the entire San Gabriel Wilderness, a panorama you'll find nowhere else.

Return to Twin Peaks Saddle, and then walk up-trail to the aforementioned junction at 8.5 miles. This time, take the right fork and climb to meet the Mount Waterman Trail coming up from Buckhorn Trailhead at 9.5 miles. Stay left and continue up to the summit of Mount Waterman, the highest point in the wilderness area, at 10.3 miles (GPS N34° 20.192' W117° 56.176'). After taking in the view (excellent but not as good as from Twin Peaks), descend the main trail to Buckhorn (see next hike).

■ Hike 51 MOUNT WATERMAN FROM BUCKHORN 🥾 🐕

HIKE LENGTH 6 miles out-and-back; 1,300' elevation gain
DIFFICULTY Moderate
SEASON June–October
MAP Tom Harrison *Angeles High Country*
PERMIT N/A

■ FEATURES

Note: This hike is within the Bobcat Fire Closure Area and is closed at least through April 1, 2022. Patches of the forest on Mount Waterman burned. Check with the U.S. Forest Service (fs.usda.gov/angeles) before visiting.

In 1889, when the San Gabriels were almost totally wild and unexplored and grizzlies frequented the area, Bob Waterman; his bride, Liz; and Commodore Perry Switzer—all of famed Switzer's Camp in the Arroyo Seco—made a three-week trip across the range to the desert and back. En route they scrambled up the highest mountain in the vicinity to get their

Hunters in Chilao backcountry (circa 1890)

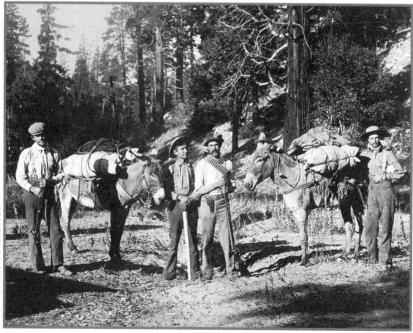

bearings. On the summit they built a cairn and left a register. In honor of Liz, who they believed to be the first white woman to cross the range, the two men christened the peak Lady Waterman Mountain. Years later, when the U.S. Geological Survey mapped the mountain, it left off the *Lady* part of the designation. Bob Waterman, who lived many years longer in Pasadena, tried several times to restore his wife's honor by putting the *Lady* back on the peak, to no avail. Today it's just Mount Waterman.

Today Mount Waterman, at 8,038 feet, is best known to skiers. Several ski lifts ascend the broad north slope of the mountain, though they are generally open only a few weekends each winter when conditions are good. In summer, when the snow is gone, Mount Waterman becomes the sole domain of the hiker. Most take this well-graded, easy-to-follow trail from Buckhorn, the shortest way up the mountain.

Waterman is an elongated, broad-summited mountain shaped like a mammoth *U*, with three high points. The southernmost of the three is the rocky highest summit. For a better view of the western San Gabriels and Devils Canyon with fewer trees in the way, walk south onto a nearby bump.

■ **DESCRIPTION**

Exit the 210 Freeway at Angeles Crest Highway (Highway 2; Exit 20) in La Cañada Flintridge. Drive 33 miles north and east to the Buckhorn Trailhead, at mile 2 LA 58.00 (GPS N34° 20.819' W117° 55.294').

From the parking area, cross over to the south side of the highway. Follow the well-graded Mount Waterman Trail—not the old roadbed that parallels the trail at first—along a shady slope. After climbing southward through tall stands of Jeffrey pines, white firs, and incense cedars for 1.1 miles, the trail reaches a saddle on Waterman's east ridge; from here you look down into the wild upper reaches of Bear Canyon and to Twin Peaks beyond. The trail now turns west and climbs to a junction with the Twin Peaks Trail at 2.1 miles. Go right and continue up to the broad, undulating summit plateau. Shortly before the peak, the trail forks. The lesser-used right fork leads to the ski area, while the left fork climbs to the high point (GPS N34° 20.192' W117° 56.176'). If you want to scramble up the summit rocks, it's easiest to circle around and ascend their west side.

Return the way you came, or make a loop by descending the ski-area service road.

▪ Hike 52 CLOUDBURST TO COOPER CANYON FALLS TO BUCKHORN 🥾 🐕 👫 🏃

HIKE LENGTH 4.5 miles one-way; 1,300' elevation loss, 800' elevation gain
DIFFICULTY Moderate
SEASON May–October
MAP Tom Harrison *Angeles High Country*
PERMIT Post Adventure Pass.

▪ FEATURES

Note: This hike is within the Bobcat Fire Closure Area and is closed at least through April 1, 2022. Patches of the forest in Cooper Canyon burned. Check with the U.S. Forest Service (fs.usda.gov/angeles) before visiting.

Beautiful, woodsy Cooper Canyon, a major tributary of Little Rock Creek, has long been a favorite of hikers. Its little singing creek, shaded by beautiful stands of Jeffrey and sugar pines, cedars, alders, and oaks, was once a favorite Native American haunt. According to mountain historian Will Thrall, braves camped at Buckhorn, just over the ridge, and sent the women and children here while the men hunted and raised a ruckus. For many years the old Native American campsite in the upper canyon, now Cooper Canyon Trail Camp, was known as Squaw Camp. The canyon became the favorite hunting ground of Pasadena brothers Ike and Tom Cooper during the 1890s, when deer and bear were plentiful. The Cooper brothers are long gone, but their exploits are eternalized by the canyon name. Part of this scenic hike lies within the new Pleasant View Ridge Wilderness, 26,752 acres set aside by Congress in 2009. No permit is required to enter.

The loop trip, requiring a shuttle between Cloudburst Summit on the Angeles Crest Highway and Buckhorn Campground, takes you down through this richly forested recess where nature's stillness reigns supreme. To make the trip more leisurely and allow time to enjoy the beauty of this canyon country, stay overnight at Cooper Canyon Trail Camp.

▪ DESCRIPTION

This hike involves a 1.5-mile car or bicycle shuttle or a risky walk along the shoulder of the Angeles Crest Highway to close the loop. To leave your getaway vehicle at Buckhorn Campground, exit the 210 Freeway at Angeles Crest Highway (Highway 2; Exit 20) in La Cañada Flintridge. Drive 34 miles north and east to the easily missed turnoff for Buckhorn Campground on the left, at mile marker 2 LA 58.25 on Angeles Crest Highway. Drive all the way through the campground to the far (northeast) end, where a short stub of dirt road leads to the Burkhart Trailhead parking area (GPS N34° 20.860' W117° 54.653'). To reach the trailhead at Cloudburst Summit, exit the campground on a one-way road that rejoins the Angeles Crest Highway. Turn right and drive west about 2 miles to Cloudburst Summit at mile marker 2 LA 57.04 (GPS N34° 21.088' W117° 56.063').

Proceed on foot past the locked gate and 1.5 miles down the fire road to Cooper Canyon Trail Camp, on a forested bench to your right (GPS N34° 21.665' W117° 55.265'). Tables, stoves, and a vault toilet make this a free and convenient first-come, first-served camping spot. Stream water is available seasonally. Take the Pacific Crest Trail (PCT) east down Cooper Canyon to its junction with the Burkhart Trail leading up to Buckhorn, at 2.8 miles.

If the creek is flowing, it's well worth a 100-yard walk east on the PCT to the top of Cooper Canyon Falls. A steep and potentially hazardous path drops to the pool at the base of the falls (GPS N34° 21.658' W117° 54.136').

Back at the junction, turn south onto the Burkhart Trail and follow it up to the Buckhorn Campground hiker's parking area. Near the top, you'll pass a 10-foot waterfall easily accessible from the trail.

VARIATION If you don't want to set up the shuttle, you can make this an out-and-back hike from Cloudburst Summit (5.5 miles) or Buckhorn Campground (3.2 miles).

■ Hike 53 WINSTON PEAK ↗ 🐕 🚶

HIKE LENGTH 1.2 miles out-and-back; 500' elevation gain
DIFFICULTY Easy
SEASON May–October
MAP Tom Harrison *Angeles High Country*
PERMIT N/A

■ FEATURES

Note: This hike is within the Bobcat Fire Closure Area and is closed at least through April 1, 2022. Winston Peak appears to have escaped the burn. Check with the U.S. Forest Service (fs.usda.gov/angeles) before visiting.

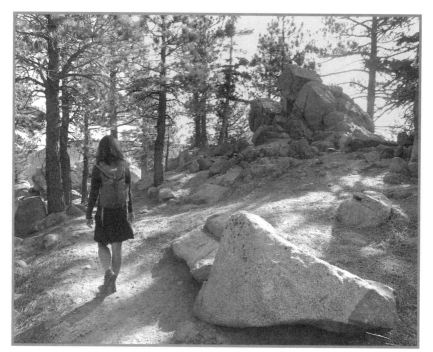

Summit rocks of Winston Peak

Winston Peak (7,502') is an appealing summit in the Pleasant View Wilderness, accessible by an easy hike through an open forest of Jeffrey pines and white firs accented by lupine and other wildflowers. Although it lacks an official trail, hikers have worn a clear and straightforward path to the summit. The trip is particularly appealing in May or June when the flowers are in peak bloom. The peak is named for L. C. Winston, a banker from Pasadena who died here in 1900 when he was caught in a blizzard while hunting.

■ DESCRIPTION

Exit the 210 Freeway at Angeles Crest Highway (Highway 2; Exit 20) in La Cañada Flintridge. Drive 34 miles north and east to Cloudburst Summit at mile marker 2 LA 57.04. Park in a turnout on the north side of the road by Forest Road 3N02 (GPS N34° 21.088' W117° 56.063').

From the parking area, FR 3N02 leads north past a gate and the PCT starts to the right, but we take an unsigned abandoned road that climbs steeply to the left instead. Within 0.1 mile join a climbers' trail on the left that shortcuts a bend in the road. Take this trail half a mile to the boulder pile on the summit of Winston Peak (GPS N34° 21.509' W117° 56.143').

VARIATION If you're looking for a longer hike with more of the same fine scenery, you can follow the climbers' trail down the far side and on to Winston Ridge, then loop back by way of the Pacific Crest Trail (PCT). This loop is 4.4 miles with 1,400 feet of elevation gain.

The climbers' trail leads down the steeper north side of Winston Peak to a saddle where you meet the PCT (GPS N34° 21.810' W117° 55.819'). Instead of taking the PCT, stay left onto another climbers' trail that circles around the west side of Peak 6,903 to a second saddle (GPS N34° 22.037' W117° 55.753'). Continue along the climbers' trail to another boulder pile on the 7,003-foot high point of Winston Ridge (GPS N34° 22.272' W117° 56.154').

When you're done, retrace your steps to the second saddle. For variety, stay left here and circle the east side of Peak 6,903 until you reach the PCT at a junction that is easily overlooked by PCT hikers (GPS N34° 21.914' W117° 55.622'). Turn right and take the PCT back to the first saddle; then follow the PCT as it contours across the east side of Winston Peak. When you reach a junction with FR 3N02, you can take either the PCT or the road to Cloudburst Summit.

■ Hike 54 PLEASANT VIEW RIDGE 🥾 🐐 🚶

HIKE LENGTH 12 miles out-and-back; 3,500' elevation gain
DIFFICULTY Strenuous
SEASON May–October
MAP Tom Harrison *Angeles High Country*
PERMIT Post Adventure Pass.

■ FEATURES

Note: This hike is within the Bobcat Fire Closure Area and is closed at least through April 1, 2022. Portions of the forest along this hike burned. Check with the U.S. Forest Service (fs.usda.gov/angeles) before visiting.

Long, sinuous Pleasant View Ridge lives up to its name. A hiker resting in the shade of tall Jeffrey pines on its crest can gaze far out into the seemingly endless Mojave Desert. On the clearest of days, you can make out the tawny, sharp-toothed ramparts of the southern Sierra Nevada

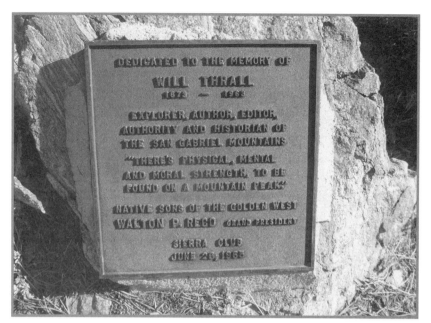

This plaque on Pleasant View Ridge commemorates Will Thrall, patron saint of Southern California hiking guidebook authors.

more than 60 miles in the distance. The area was designated as wilderness in 2009, preserving 26,752 acres in their natural, wild state. No permit is required to enter.

Looking at Pleasant View Ridge from the Angeles Crest Highway, you may think that it is close at hand. But it's farther than you realize. Separating the ridge from the main body of the range is the V-shaped trench of Little Rock Creek, a desert-bound creek whose canyon holds sylvan surprises where you might least expect to find them. To reach Pleasant View, you must descend into the deep canyon and climb up the other side.

Be in shape for this one. It's down and up both ways, with little level going. If the day is warm, carry plenty of water. You could spend a peaceful night on the summit if you have enough water.

■ DESCRIPTION

Exit the 210 Freeway at Angeles Crest Highway (Highway 2; Exit 20) in La Cañada Flintridge. Drive 34 miles north and east to the easily missed turn-off for Buckhorn Campground on the left, at mile 58.25. Drive all the way through the campground to the far (northeast) end, where a short stub of dirt road leads to the Burkhart Trailhead parking area (GPS N34° 20.860' W117° 54.653').

Follow the Burkhart Trail 1.6 miles down to Cooper Canyon. Along the way, you'll pass a 10-foot waterfall easily accessible from the trail and may hear a 30-foot waterfall farther down that is unsafe to try to reach.

At the canyon floor, turn right on the Pacific Crest Trail. Follow it past beautiful Cooper Canyon Falls; a steep and possibly dangerous path drops to the pool at the base. At 1.8 miles, turn left to leave the PCT and rejoin another part of the Burkhart Trail that steadily climbs around a ridge, crosses a small creek (flowing in spring and early summer), and zigzags up 1,300 feet to Burkhart Saddle at 4.9 miles (6,959'; GPS N34° 23.125' W117° 53.643').

If you are weary, this is a good turnaround point. Otherwise, find an unmarked climbers trail leading west up the steep slope. Climb over Will Thrall Peak (5.4 miles, 7,845'; GPS N34° 23.066' W117° 54.151'), named for the historian, conservationist, and pioneering guidebook author who founded *Trails Magazine* in the 1930s. Continue northwest through Jeffrey pines to the 7,983-foot high point of Pleasant View Ridge at 5.9 miles (GPS N34° 23.397' W117° 54.554'), a 1,000-foot elevation gain from the saddle. From here the view is outstanding. Return the way you came.

VARIATION You can descend the desert side of the Burkhart Trail 7 miles to Devil's Punchbowl (see Hike 59), if you arrange a long car shuttle.

■ **Hike 55 EAGLES ROOST PICNIC AREA TO COOPER CANYON FALLS** ↗ 🐕

HIKE LENGTH 7 miles out-and-back; 1,100' elevation gain
DIFFICULTY Moderate
SEASON May–October
MAP Tom Harrison *Angeles High Country*
PERMIT Post Adventure Pass, or park outside fee area.

■ **FEATURES**

Note: This hike is within the Bobcat Fire Closure Area and is closed at least through April 1, 2022. Portions of the forest along this hike burned. Check with the U.S. Forest Service (fs.usda.gov/angeles) before visiting.

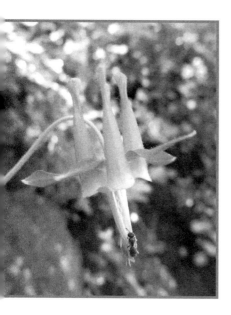

Brilliant orange-and-yellow columbine flowers favor moist areas, including Cooper Canyon Falls.

Note: Since 2005, the portion of Little Rock Creek described in this trip has been closed to protect the habitat of the endangered mountain yellow-legged frog. Because the Forest Service plans to reopen this excellent trail, I've left it in the book. Check with the Forest Service before your trip to see if it has reopened. If this route is closed, use Hike 52 to visit Cooper Canyon Falls instead.

Some of the most magnificent canyon country in the San Gabriel Mountains lies on the desert slopes of the range. Nowhere is this more evident than in the uppermost reaches of Little Rock Creek, close under Kratka Ridge and Mount Williamson's southwest shoulder. The terrain is rugged and colorful—sheer crags of whitish rock stand in stark contrast to wrinkled slopes of reddish brown and gray. Jeffrey, sugar, and Coulter pines, as well as white firs, incense cedars, and oaks, crowd canyon recesses and dot open ridges. The delightful stream, fed by springs high in the granite folds of Mount Williamson, runs all year.

This trip leaves the Angeles Crest Highway opposite Eagles Roost Picnic Area and descends the Pacific Crest Trail (PCT) into the upper reaches of Little Rock Creek. Once you leave the highway, you drop into recesses as magnificently wild as any in the range. If you like primitive canyon country undisturbed by civilization, this hike should be a rewarding experience. The entire surrounding area north of the highway was officially declared a wilderness area in 2009.

■ DESCRIPTION

Exit the 210 Freeway at Angeles Crest Highway (Highway 2; Exit 20) in La Cañada Flintridge. Drive 37 miles north and east to the Eagles Roost Picnic Area at mile marker 2 LA 61.65 (GPS N34° 21.264' W117° 52.690').

Cross the highway and descend west on the PCT into the head of Little Rock Creek, reaching the bottom in a mile. Here, amid a darkened forest and alongside the cold waters of the creek, you will be tempted to pause. Back on the main route, follow the trail as it contours along the north slope of the gorge, heading downstream (west). You round rocky points, with the creek far below, and pass through sheltered recesses, then drop down alongside the creek and reach a junction with the Burkhart Trail on the right, leading to Burkhart Saddle at 3.3 miles (see previous hike). Continue 0.2 mile on the PCT to Cooper Canyon Falls, which you can view from the trail (GPS N34° 21.658' W117° 54.136'). A steep and possibly dangerous path descends to a pool at the base. Return the way you came.

VARIATIONS You can make this a great 5-mile one-way trip with a 3.5-mile car or bicycle shuttle by continuing just past Cooper Canyon Falls and turning left onto the Burkhart Trail, which climbs to Buckhorn Campground (see Hike 52).

■ Hike 56 MOUNT WILLIAMSON ↗ 🐕 🚶

HIKE LENGTH 3.6 miles out-and-back; 1,400' elevation gain
DIFFICULTY Moderate
SEASON June–October
MAP Tom Harrison *Angeles High Country*
PERMIT N/A

■ FEATURES

Note: This hike is within the Bobcat Fire Closure Area and is closed at least through April 1, 2022. Patches of forest on Mount Williamson burned. Check with the U.S. Forest Service (fs.usda.gov/angeles) before visiting.

Mount Williamson, all 8,214 feet of it, stands tall and massive, jutting northward from the main crest of the range like a bold sentinel guarding the green high country from the withering influence of the desert 5,000 feet below. It is buttressed to the south by formidable cliffs, through which the Angeles Crest Highway tunnels. To the north, it plunges abruptly down to that fantastic jumble of whitish rocks known as the Devil's Punchbowl.

The mountain is named for Lieutenant Robert Stockton Williamson of the U.S. Army, who led a reconnaissance of the north slopes of the

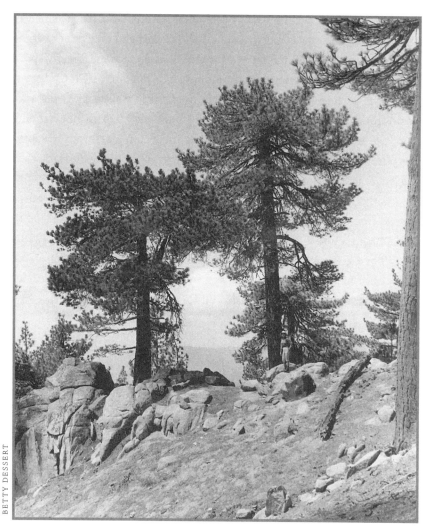

BETTY DESSERT

High on Mount Williamson Ridge

San Gabriels for the Pacific Railroad Survey in 1853. He was looking for a railway route across the mountains. (Williamson succeeded, locating *two* railway routes across the mountains—Soledad Pass and Cajon Pass.) The report he submitted to Congress contained the first detailed description of the desert side of the range.

From the summit of Mount Williamson, you get an eagle's-eye view of the broken country explored by this Army officer more than a century ago. It has changed much, but the strange geological features—scarps; beeline valleys; troughs; sag ponds; and, most of all, the twisted and folded rocks of the Devil's Punchbowl—are the same. Mount Williamson towers directly above the San Andreas Rift Zone, the most monumental fault in the United States. Its unique pattern is readily observable to any who walk a short distance north from the summit and look down. The fault line can be seen extending along the entire northern base of the San Gabriels, from northwest to southeast. Only from Mount Williamson or from high points along Pleasant View Ridge, immediately to the northwest, do you get this perspective.

Although you're in the Pleasant View Ridge Wilderness, no permit is needed. You could spend a starry night on the summit if you make sure to haul enough water.

If you go in April or May, you will likely encounter Pacific Crest Trail (PCT) thru-hikers on their pilgrimage from Mexico to Canada. Consider being a trail angel by bringing fresh fruit for these shaggy trekkers.

■ DESCRIPTION

Exit the 210 Freeway at Angeles Crest Highway (Highway 2; Exit 20) in La Cañada Flintridge. Drive 38 miles north and east to the large, north-side turnout at mile 2 LA 62.50 (GPS N34° 21.712' W117° 52.200').

From the large turnout, take the PCT at the east end of the parking area that switchbacks up Williamson's southwest ridge. You pass through an open forest of Jeffrey and ponderosa pines, with white firs becoming more abundant as you near 8,000 feet. In 1.5 miles you reach the ridgetop, where the Pacific Crest Trail begins descending toward Islip Saddle. From this point you are rewarded with a superb view southward, directly into the rugged trench of Bear Canyon, 3,000 feet below. To reach the summit, leave the PCT and follow a less-used trail northward along the ridge, climbing to the 8,214-foot high point overlooking the desert at 1.8 miles (GPS N34° 22.265' W117° 51.497'). This point is shown as the summit on the topo map, although a bump 0.25 mile northwest is 30 feet higher and offers a better view of the Devil's Punchbowl country.

VARIATION You can also climb Mount Williamson from Islip Saddle, 1.6 miles east of the trailhead recommended above. The route is approximately the same distance and elevation gain. With a 1.5-mile car or bicycle shuttle, you can make it an enjoyable point-to-point hike.

■ Hike 57 WILLIAMSON–BURKHART TRAVERSE

HIKE LENGTH 12-mile loop; 3,500' elevation gain
DIFFICULTY Strenuous
SEASON June–October
MAP Tom Harrison *Angeles High Country*
PERMIT N/A

■ FEATURES

Note: This hike is within the Bobcat Fire Closure Area and is closed at least through April 1, 2022. Patches of forest in this area burned. Check with the U.S. Forest Service (fs.usda.gov/angeles) before visiting.

Note: Since 2005, the U.S. Forest Service has closed the portion of Little Rock Creek described in this trip, to protect the habitat of the endangered mountain yellow-legged frog. As of 2018, the Forest Service was considering mitigations to allow reopening the trail. Check with them before attempting this trip. An alternate exit route is described below.

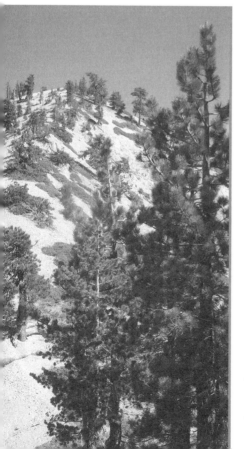

This is a long up-and-down ramble over the northern crest of the San Gabriels, partly on trail, partly cross-country, through the Pleasant View Ridge Wilderness (no permit required). The trip features a trailless traverse along the rim of Pleasant View Ridge between Mount Williamson and Burkhart Saddle, with continuous views over desert and high mountain country. It is a tough but rewarding experience for those in top physical condition.

A climbers' trail follows the ridge between Mount Williamson and Burkhart Saddle

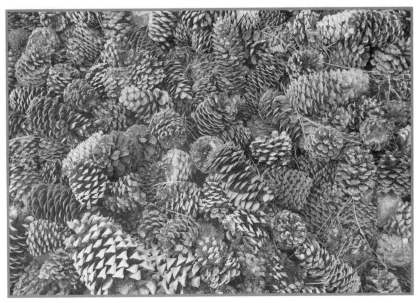

Jeffrey and sugar pine cones on Pleasant View Ridge

Don't try it alone; much of the terrain is seldom trod by human feet, and rescue would be difficult. Carry all the water you need; most of the route is waterless. There are flat spots along the ridge where you could find dispersed dry camping, but hauling an overnight pack might be harder than doing this as a day hike.

■ DESCRIPTION

Exit the 210 Freeway at Angeles Crest Highway (Highway 2; Exit 20) in La Cañada Flintridge. Drive 38 miles north and east to the large, north-side turnout at mile 2 LA 62.50 (GPS N34° 21.712' W117° 52.200').

Take the Pacific Crest Trail (PCT) 1.5 miles onto the shoulder of Mount Williamson. Turn left and follow the summit trail to the second, higher summit (see previous hike) of Mount Williamson at 2.1 miles. When the maintained trail ends at the summit, walk northwest along the top of Pleasant View Ridge. You might see glints from an aircraft wreck on a ridge across Holcomb Canyon to the north. In 1.1 miles, the ridge bends to the right. An optional side trip 0.5 mile to the northeast brings you to the crash site (GPS N34° 23.142' W117° 51.917'), where a C-119 Flying Boxcar from March Field crashed in 1966 on a routine training mission. Our main route turns west and descends to a saddle, then climbs back over Pallet Mountain (4.2 miles, 7,760'; GPS N34° 23.154' W117° 53.156') before dropping down to Burkhart Saddle at (4.8 miles, 6,959'). This cross-country jaunt is open, through a rich forest of Jeffrey pines, but the steep up-and-down is tiring. Rest often and enjoy the superb desert view, with occasional glimpses down into the heart of the Devil's Punchbowl.

From Burkhart Saddle, turn left (south) and follow the Burkhart Trail down to Little Rock Creek (see Hike 54), where you meet the PCT at 8.3 miles. At the time of this writing, the eastbound segment is closed to protect frog habitat. If it has reopened, you can follow it 3.3 miles up to the Angeles Crest Highway opposite Eagles Roost Picnic Area (see Hike 55). Walk northeast on the highway or along the PCT 0.9 mile to your car.

An alternative, if the PCT to Eagles Roost is still off-limits, is to jog west on the PCT 0.2 mile, passing Cooper Canyon Falls, and then turn south onto another portion of the Burkhart Trail that climbs to Buckhorn Campground (see Hike 52). This option shaves off 1.6 miles of hiking but requires a 4-mile bicycle or car shuttle.

VARIATION From Burkhart Saddle, you could extend this trip by climbing west to Will Thrall Peak and Pleasant View Ridge (see Hike 54) or by descending the Burkhart Trail to the Devil's Punchbowl (Hike 59).

■ Hike 58 KRATKA RIDGE 🥾 🐕 🚶

HIKE LENGTH 1.8 miles out-and-back; 400' elevation gain
DIFFICULTY Easy
SEASON June–November
MAP Tom Harrison *Angeles High Country*
PERMIT Post Adventure Pass, or park outside fee area.

■ FEATURES

Note: This hike is within the Bobcat Fire Closure Area and is closed at least through April 1, 2022. Patches of forest on Kratka Ridge burned. Check with the U.S. Forest Service (fs.usda.gov/angeles) before visiting.

You won't find more-outstanding views per step traveled along the Pacific Crest Trail (PCT) in the San Gabriel Mountains than you do on Kratka Ridge. This easy stretch of the trail is routed on the breathtaking ridge overlooking the upper reaches of Bear Creek in the San Gabriel

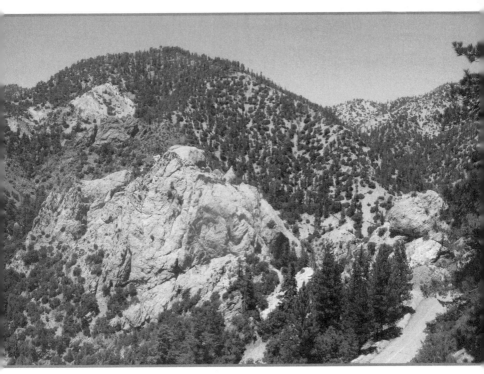

Williamson Rock from Kratka Ridge

Wilderness. The ridge is named for George and Walter Kratka of Pasadena. Don't confuse this hike with the nearby Kratka Ridge/Snowcrest ski area on Mount Waterman.

■ DESCRIPTION

Exit the 210 Freeway at Angeles Crest Highway (Highway 2; Exit 20) in La Cañada Flintridge. Drive 37 miles north and east to the Eagles Roost Picnic Area at mile marker 2 LA 61.65 (GPS N34° 21.264' W117° 52.690').

From the picnic area, follow the PCT northeast as it briefly parallels the highway before climbing onto Kratka Ridge. The first part of the ridge has out-of-place Coulter pines that were apparently planted here; farther along, expect Jeffrey and sugar pines. Look for Williamson Rock hulking across the canyon to the north. The popular rock-climbing area and adjacent portion of the PCT have been closed by the U.S. Forest Service since 2005 to protect the endangered mountain yellow-legged frog.

The trail stays high for 0.9 mile before dropping to meet the highway again at mile 2 LA 62.50 (GPS N34° 21.712' W117° 52.200'). If you left a bicycle shuttle here, you can pedal back. Otherwise, turn around and retrace your steps to enjoy the view in the opposite direction. Walking back on the shoulder of the busy highway could be dangerous.

■ Hike 59 BURKHART TRAIL ↗ 🐕

HIKE LENGTH 14 miles out-and-back; 3,200' elevation gain
DIFFICULTY Strenuous
SEASON October–June
MAP Tom Harrison *Angeles High Country*
PERMIT N/A (free parking at Punchbowl)

■ FEATURES

Note: This hike is within the Bobcat Fire Closure Area and is closed at least through April 1, 2022. The desert slopes north of Burkhart Saddle burned severely. Check with the Forest Service (fs.usda.gov/angeles) before visiting.

South from Littlerock and Pearblossom, several rounded ridgelines rise rather abruptly from the desert. Most prominent of these is Pleasant View Ridge, a long, sinuous hogback that begins its upward trend near Juniper Hills, leads southeasterly, and reaches its climax at 8,214-foot Mount Williamson. The ridge is aptly named. A hiker resting atop one of its many welts can look down upon little valleys and low foothills resplendent with the Mojave's best-known symbol: the beautiful Joshua tree, sharing the landscape with clusters of mesquite, purple sage, and yucca. In springtime, after abundant rain, the foothills are carpeted with colorful wildflowers. Hardy junipers and piñons dot the higher slopes. And in the distance, beyond the strange wrinkles of the San Andreas Fault, the Mojave Desert sprawls far and wide.

The Burkhart Trail, built years ago by a rancher of that name, is the only maintained footpath onto Pleasant View Ridge. The trail ascends the steep west slopes of Cruthers Creek from the desert to Burkhart Saddle, a distinct gap on the crest between Will Thrall Peak and Pallett Mountain. Except in a few places, it is gently graded as it climbs steadily from Joshua trees and sages through a piñon forest, and finally into Jeffrey-pine country along the ridgetop.

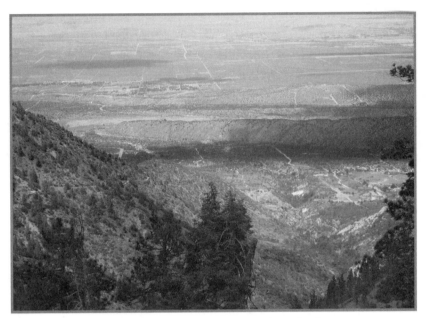

The Burkhart Trail descends from Burkhart Saddle to the desert.

The Burkhart Trail is a fitting introduction to the desert side of the San Gabriels, a side not well known to most Southern California hikers.

■ **DESCRIPTION**

From the Antelope Valley Freeway (Highway 14) south of Palmdale, exit at Pearblossom Highway (Highway 138; Exit 35). Follow Pearblossom Highway east 14 miles to the small community of Pearblossom. At Pearblossom, turn right (south) on Longview Road (County Road N6) at a sign for Devil's Punchbowl. In 2.3 miles, turn left on Fort Cajon Road. In 0.3 mile, turn right to stay on CR N6, and follow the twisting road 5.3 miles to its end at the Punchbowl (GPS N34° 24.841' W117° 51.468').

Walk south from the nature center, and pick up the trail as it passes behind a metal water tank and veers right at a junction (0.8 mile) signed BURKHART SADDLE 6.2 MILES. Follow the trail as it contours the mountain slope through Jeffrey pines and manzanitas. You drop into Cruthers Creek at 3.4 miles and then climb the west slope and traverse upward high above the creek through piñons. You pass a small spring (dependable only in rainy season) and finally reach Burkhart Saddle at 6.8 miles (GPS N34°

23.125' W117° 53.643'), from which you look down into Little Rock Creek. Return the way you came.

VARIATIONS If you have energy to spare, you can climb a faint trail leading right (west) up Pleasant View Ridge, around Will Thrall Peak, ending on a small flat on the crest (1 mile and 1,000' of gain from the saddle, see Hike 54. Or you can descend south from Burkhart Saddle into Little Rock Creek and on up to Buckhorn on the Angeles Crest Highway (12 miles from the Punchbowl to Buckhorn with a long car shuttle; also see Hike 54). Another option is to continue east, on your return, via the High Desert Trail across the top of Devil's Punchbowl past Devils Chair to South Fork Campground (see Hike 61).

■ Hike 60 DEVIL'S PUNCHBOWL NATURAL AREA AND NATURE CENTER ◗ 🐕 👫

HIKE LENGTH 1.2-mile loop; 300' elevation gain and loss
DIFFICULTY Easy
SEASON October–June
MAP Tom Harrison *Angeles High Country*
PERMIT N/A (free parking at Punchbowl)

■ FEATURES

Note: This hike is within the Bobcat Fire Closure Area and is closed at least through April 1, 2022. Devil's Punchbowl burned severely. The Nature Center was destroyed, and the county park is closed until further notice; check the website (parks.lacounty.gov) before visiting.

The great San Andreas Rift Zone cuts a beeline swath along the desert side of the San Gabriels. Many interesting geological features lie along this monumental earthquake fault system, but none so strange as the fantastic jumble of whitish rocks known as the Devil's Punchbowl. Within this mile-wide depression rise row upon row of weathered sandstone blocks, many of them tilted so as to resemble plates standing on edge, others folded and broken like huge slices of fancy pudding.

In 1963 this unique geological formation became a Los Angeles County park. A paved road was built on its western rim, and a wide, well-graded loop trail was hacked out down into the bowl.

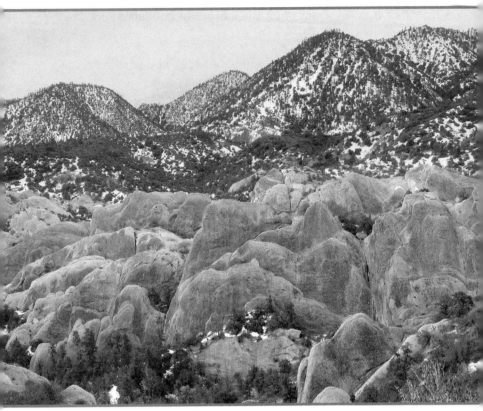

Devil's Punchbowl is a unique feature on the San Andreas Fault Rift Zone.

Although only a short down-and-up walk, this otherworldly loop trip into the Devil's Punchbowl is one of the most interesting treks in the range. The trail passes beside weird sandstone outcrops, and at the bottom of the bowl, a playful stream cascades over, around, and through the slanted formations. Hardy piñons and manzanita thickets cling to precipitous footholds between the rocks.

■ DESCRIPTION

From the Antelope Valley Freeway (Highway 14) south of Palmdale, exit at Pearblossom Highway (Highway 138; Exit 35). Follow Pearblossom Highway east 14 miles to the small community of Pearblossom. At Pearblossom, turn right (south) on Longview Road (County Road N6) at a sign for the Devil's Punchbowl. In 2.3 miles, turn left on Fort Cajon Road. In 0.3 mile, turn right to stay on CR N6, and follow the twisting road 5.3 miles to its end at the Punchbowl (GPS N34° 24.841' W117° 51.468'). The park is open sunrise–sunset; parking is free.

From the parking area, walk east past the park headquarters (which has restrooms, picnic tables, and interpretive displays) to the well-marked beginning of the trail. Follow the trail as it winds 300 feet down into the Punchbowl, turns right just above the bottom, and then ascends back up to the parking area. The trail is gently graded for the most part (one short, steep pitch on the way out), and it is well worth the stride down and the huff-and-puff back out just to see firsthand what nature, in a fit of originality, has wrought.

■ Hike 61 DEVILS CHAIR ↗ 🐕 👫 🏃

HIKE LENGTH 5.5 miles out-and-back; 1,300' elevation gain
DIFFICULTY Moderate
SEASON October–June
MAP Tom Harrison *Angeles High Country*
PERMIT N/A

■ FEATURES

Note: This hike is within the Bobcat Fire Closure Area and is closed at least through April 1, 2022. This area burned severely. Check with the U.S. Forest Service (fs.usda.gov/angeles) before visiting.

This trip climbs over a ridge and enters the "back door" of Devil's Punchbowl. It visits the wilder eastern part of the jumbled depression, a section not reached by the loop trail from county park headquarters (see previous hike). It takes you to the strangest, most unique formation in the Punchbowl—the huge white-rock mass, sheer on three sides, known as the Devils Chair. Those with vivid imaginations can make out the devil himself sitting on his throne, lording over his topsy-turvy domain.

■ DESCRIPTION

From Highway 138, 26.5 miles northwest of I-15 or 16.7 miles east of Highway 14, turn south on 165th Street. Follow the meandering road 6.4 miles as its name changes to Bob's Gap Road. Turn left on County Road N4 (Big Pines Highway), go 0.3 mile, and then turn right on Big Rock

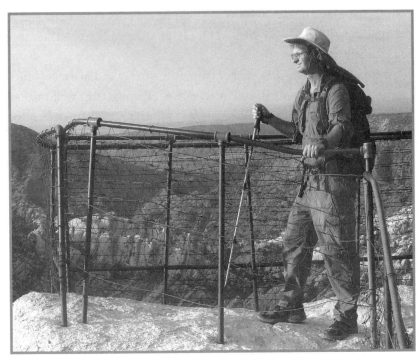

The Devils Chair is an airy perch overlooking the Punchbowl.

Creek Road and go 2.4 miles. Turn right onto graded Forest Road 4N11A and proceed 0.9 mile to South Fork Campground. Just before the campground entrance, look for the signed Manzanita Trail on the left. Opposite this sign, take a short dirt spur on the right to the trailhead parking (GPS N34° 23.832' W117° 49.350').

Walk south from the parking lot, pick up the trail, and follow it south about 50 yards to a junction, where you turn right (west), cross the boulder-strewn creekbed, and climb through piñons, scrub oaks, manzanitas, and mountain mahoganies to a saddle on the ridge at 1.2 miles. You contour and then drop into Holcomb Canyon. Here you find a rare meeting of three plant communities: pine, piñon/juniper, and streamside woodland. By late spring the yuccas are in full bloom. The trail fords tiny Holcomb Creek near a secluded campsite at 2.1 miles (seasonal water) and then zigzags over another ridge, skirting the upper section of the devil's domain. At 2.6 miles, you reach a short side trail leading onto the huge rock promontory known as the Devils Chair, where you have a breathtaking view of the Punchbowl

(GPS N34° 24.148' W117° 50.737'). If you venture onto the Devils Chair, stay within the protective fence. Return the way you came.

VARIATION An attractive option is to continue west on the High Desert Trail, traversing the forest-clad slopes above the Punchbowl, to the Burkhart Trail connection, and turn north on the latter down to park headquarters at 6 miles. You need a car shuttle for this (see Hike 59).

▪ Hike 62 SOUTH FORK TRAIL 🥾 🐐

HIKE LENGTH 10 miles out-and-back; 2,100' elevation gain
DIFFICULTY Moderate
SEASON All year (upper part may be snowbound after winter storms)
MAP Tom Harrison *Angeles High Country*
PERMIT N/A

▪ FEATURES

Note: This hike is within the Bobcat Fire Closure Area and is closed at least through April 1, 2022. Patches of forest burned along this hike. Check with

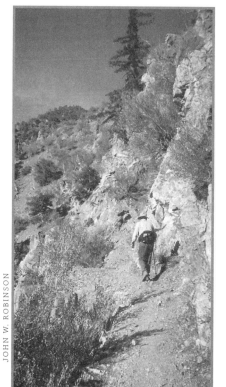

JOHN W. ROBINSON

the U.S. Forest Service (fs.usda.gov /angeles) before visiting.

The north face of the San Gabriel Mountains rises abruptly out of the desert, especially the parts along the middle and eastern high country. Some of the canyons that incise this rampart are quite imposing, being deep, V-shaped gorges. Probably the most impressive of these north-facing canyons is the South Fork of Big Rock Creek, which carves a steep path as it drops from high on the Angeles Crest down into the San Andreas Rift region at the foot of the mountains.

Ascending South Fork Trail

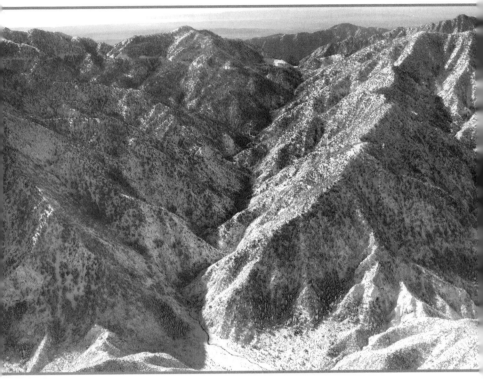

Aerial view up South Fork to Islip Saddle after a winter storm. Mount Islip (left) and Mount Williamson (right) flank the saddle.

An old trail—once a major route into the high country, before the Angeles Crest Highway forever changed the face of the mountains—climbs upcanyon all the way from South Fork Campground to Islip Saddle, passing from piñons to pines, from sages to snowbrushes, from cacti to ceanothus. The trail is seldom trod nowadays, for it culminates at the aforementioned busy transmountain thoroughfare. But its lower and middle parts hold appeal—the flora is a curious blend of desert and alpine, and the landscape is often more vertical than horizontal. Some parts of the trail cling to cliff edges, and others are covered in a slough of scree, so this is a trail for the surefooted.

■ DESCRIPTION

From Highway 138, 26.5 miles northwest of I-15 or 16.7 miles east of Highway 14, turn south on 165th Street. Follow the meandering road 6.4 miles as its name changes to Bob's Gap Road. Turn left on County Road N4 (Big Pines Highway), go 0.3 mile, and then turn right on Big Rock Creek Road and go 2.4 miles. Turn right onto graded Forest Road 4N11A and proceed 0.9 mile to South Fork Campground. Just before the campground entrance, look for the signed Manzanita Trail on the left. Opposite this sign, take a short dirt spur on the right to the trailhead parking (GPS N34° 23.832' W117° 49.350').

Walk south from the parking area on the well-marked trail, going left at a junction with the trail to Devil's Punchbowl, passing South Fork Campground on your left, and entering the deep canyon of Big Rock Creek's South Fork. Follow the trail upcanyon, through cottonwoods, oaks, maples, and alders, alongside the boulder-strewn streambed.

After 0.25 mile the trail crosses to the west bank and begins climbing the canyon slopes, through scattered piñon pines. Piñons soon give way to Jeffrey pines as you climb higher, with the bubbling creek far down to your left. At 4.1 miles, you pass the trickling Reed Spring before climbing the last mile to the parking area alongside the Angeles Crest Highway at Islip Saddle (GPS N34° 21.421' W117° 51.089').

Unless you have set up a long car shuttle or plan a much longer loop hike over Mount Baden-Powell and down the Manzanita Trail (see Hike 64), return the way you came.

■ Hike 63 MANZANITA TRAIL 🏃 🐕

HIKE LENGTH 11 miles out-and-back; 2,400' elevation gain
DIFFICULTY Moderate
SEASON All year (upper part may be snowbound after winter storms)
MAP Tom Harrison *Angeles High Country*
PERMIT N/A

■ FEATURES

The northern side of the San Gabriel Mountains differs markedly from the southern side, which is more familiar to most hikers. The plant communities range from cottonwood-lined streams near the desert floor to forested canyon slopes covered with piñon pines, oaks, and manzanitas to the pine- and fir-forested peaks of the middle high country. Winter snows linger far longer on these north-facing, shady slopes than they do on the southern exposure visible from the Los Angeles area. Two huge tectonic plates, the Pacific Plate and the North American Plate, collide here, the incredible pressure forcing the mountains ever higher and resulting in a variety of interesting geological features, most notably the strange, fantastic jumble of Devil's Punchbowl County Park (see Hikes 60 and 61).

This scenic trip follows the Punchbowl Fault, an inactive strand of the great San Andreas Fault, and passes through several areas where you can see

The Manzanita Trail follows the linear Punchbowl Fault, which is prominent in this aerial view.

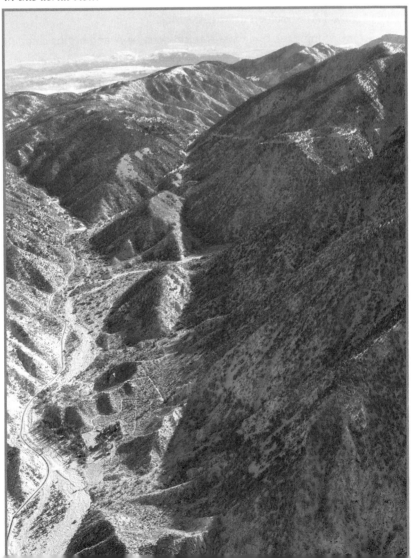

the juxtaposition of different types of rock on either side of the fault trace. It contours along the shady, north-facing slopes high above Big Rock Creek through a mixed forest of oaks; big-cone Douglas-firs; and, higher up, Jeffrey pines and white firs. It is a superb fall hike, when the air is cool and refreshing and the brilliant leaves of cottonwoods, maples, and black oaks provide a vivid contrast to the dull green and brown background.

■ DESCRIPTION

From Highway 138, 26.5 miles northwest of I-15 or 16.7 miles east of Highway 14, turn south on 165th Street. Follow the meandering road 6.4 miles as its name changes to Bob's Gap Road. Turn left on County Road N4 (Big Pines Highway), go 0.3 mile, and then turn right on Big Rock Creek Road and go 2.4 miles. Turn right onto graded Forest Road 4N11A and proceed 0.9 mile to South Fork Campground. Just before the campground entrance, look for the signed Manzanita Trail on the left. Opposite this sign, take a short dirt spur on the right to the trailhead parking (GPS N34° 23.832' W117° 49.350').

The signed Manzanita Trailhead is across the road, directly opposite the entrance to the parking area. Follow the narrow pathway as it switchbacks south up through a forest of oaks, manzanitas, and big-cone Douglas-firs 0.8 mile to a junction with a spur trail on a sandstone outcrop, and stay right on the Manzanita Trail. Continue along the trail, climbing steadily eastward, with the broad canyon of Big Rock Creek visible to your left; past a variety of interesting rock formations created by the fault; and across several small tributary canyons. At 2.9 miles, the trail descends slightly to reach the rock-strewn wash of Dorr Canyon sweeping down from your right. You may lose the trail as you scramble several hundred yards across the canyon bottom, but you should regain it on the other side as it continues up a narrow valley and across another tributary featuring a small waterfall before finally arriving at 6,565-foot Vincent Gap, 5.6 miles from the trailhead (GPS N34° 22.394' W117° 45.141'). Return the way you came.

VARIATIONS If you still have some gas left in your tank when you reach Vincent Gap, you can cross the highway and take the easy 4-mile round-trip stroll to Big Horn Mine and back (see Hike 75) and then return down to the trailhead, a total distance of 15 miles.

You can make a two-day backpack and drop down into the upper East Fork country all the way to the East Fork Trailhead (see Hike 78)—a remarkable 22-mile transit across nearly the entire range.

■ Hike 64 HIGH DESERT LOOP ◯ 🐕 🏃

HIKE LENGTH 23-mile loop; 5,500' elevation gain
DIFFICULTY Strenuous
SEASON May–November
MAP Tom Harrison *Angeles High Country*
PERMIT N/A

■ FEATURES

Note: This hike is within the Bobcat Fire Closure Area and is closed at least through April 1, 2022. Patches of forest burned along the route, particularly from Windy Gap to Islip Saddle and down the South Fork Trail. Check with the U.S. Forest Service (fs.usda.gov/angeles) before visiting.

The High Desert National Recreation Trail is the name given in 1981 to the Burkhart, Devil's Punchbowl, Manzanita, and South Fork Trails that climb the northern flank of the San Gabriel Mountains between the Mojave Desert and the Pacific Crest Trail (PCT). In combination with the PCT, these trails form a splendid loop touring many ecological zones as you climb from the desert to the highest ridges. This loop has a diversity of conifers that is unsurpassed along any trail in Southern California and is a marvelous place to learn the trees of the Angeles. Peak baggers will enjoy short detours to climb peaks along the Angeles Crest. If you do this hike in the summer, get an early start to climb out of the desert before the heat of the day. The Angeles Crest can be icy December–April.

Water may be a concern on this trail. Little Jimmy Spring is the only reliable year-round source. Lamel Spring and Reed Spring may have water in spring and summer, or all year in a wet year. In a dry fall, consider caching water at Vincent Gap and/or Islip Saddle, especially if you're leading a youth group that can't haul much water.

■ DESCRIPTION

From Highway 138, 26.5 miles northwest of I-15 or 16.7 miles east of Highway 14, turn south on 165th Street. Follow the meandering road 6.4 miles as its name changes to Bob's Gap Road. Turn left on County Road N4 (Big Pines Highway), go 0.3 mile, and then turn right on Big Rock Creek Road and go 2.4 miles. Turn right onto graded Forest Road 4N11A and proceed 0.9 mile to South Fork Campground. Just before the campground entrance, look for the signed Manzanita Trail on the left. Opposite this sign, take a short dirt spur on the right to the trailhead parking (GPS N34° 23.832' W117° 49.350').

Start your trip on the signed Manzanita Trail back on the campground road (see previous hike). This attractive but poorly named trail leads through scrub oak and birch-leaf mountain mahogany but passes very little manzanita in its entire length. The trail makes four switchbacks to climb around a sandstone outcrop. At the first switchback, you'll encounter a stand of trees, mostly big-cone Douglas-fir and canyon live oak, which are codominant for the next 3 miles.

Big-cone Douglas-fir is a conifer with rows of needles on all sides of the twigs. The cones are generally 4–6 inches long, big compared only to the ordinary Douglas-firs that grow in the Sierra and northward. Nearly all the oaks along the trail are canyon live oaks, with large acorns; flat elliptical leaves that remain on the tree year-round; and, often, many trunks from a common root. The acorns were favored by Native Americans, who harvested up to 400 pounds per tree; soaked the kernels to leach out the bitter tannins; ground them into flour using bedrock mortars called metates; and cooked them into soup, mush, biscuits, or bread. This forest community is also associated with gnats, which don't bite but love to swarm in hikers' faces.

At 0.8 mile pass a short spur to the sandstone outcrop. It's worth walking 100 yards out to the rocks to take in the view. From here, the trail climbs at a steady grade. At 1.8 miles pass another trail descending to Paradise Springs, a private camp. Continue over a small saddle and across often-dry Big Rock Creek in Dorr Canyon at 2.9 miles. After another small saddle, pass a smaller but more reliable creek decorated with wildflowers, including scarlet monkey flower and columbine. The trail follows the linear Punchbowl Fault, and the saddles are created by the fault.

Soon you'll catch the sights and sounds of the Angeles Crest Highway bridging the canyon above. Watch for a striking yellow flower called blazing star, uncommon in Southern California. Observe the forest transition to white fir, Jeffrey and sugar pine, and incense cedar before reaching Vincent

Gap at 5.6 miles. White fir has individual needles in rows. The green cones grow upright at the tops of the trees and are rarely seen on the ground. Mistletoe infests many of the white firs in this area. Jeffrey pine has long needles in bundles of three and shapely 4- to 8-inch cones. Sugar pines have short needles in bundles of five and skinny cones of 12 inches or more in length; they often drip with sugary sap. Incense cedar has bright-green scales rather than needles, ropy bark, and small seedpods rather than pine cones.

Cross the Angeles Crest Highway to a large and busy parking area at Vincent Gap (mile marker 2 LA 74.88; GPS N34° 22.394' W117° 45.141'). A picnic bench is shaded by a grove of non-native sequoias. Several trails depart the gap; be sure you take the PCT toward Mount Baden-Powell. This trail makes 40 switchbacks on its way up the mountain, which is named for Lord Robert Baden-Powell, the British lieutenant general who founded the Boy Scouts Association in 1910. At the 14th switchback (7.3 miles), a signed spur leads to Lamel Spring in a ravine (GPS N34° 22.057' W117° 45.418'), but don't rely on water here unless you have recent reports that it is running (check pctwater.com; see part 2 at mile 375.9). The switchbacks become longer. Watch for undeveloped campsites near the 17th and 20th switchbacks. By the 17th, the forest becomes almost a pure stand of lodgepole pines. These pines, which have thin, flaky bark; needles in bundles of two; and round, golf ball–size cones, are found only at high elevations in Southern California. At the 21st switchback, you'll meet two gnarled limber pines beside the trail. These pines have short needles in bundles of five on flexible twigs resembling bottlebrushes. The cones are longer, 3–6 inches, and resemble small sugar-pine cones. The bark is thicker, and the trees, which live for more than 1,000 years, are often twisted by wind and ice into fantastic shapes. Limber pines, found only on the highest summits in Southern California, mingle with the lodgepoles the rest of the way up the mountain.

The switchbacks abruptly tighten, until they stop after number 38 and you get great views along the upper ridge. Reach a trail junction beside the Wally Waldron Tree, a 1,500-year-old limber pine named for a Boy Scout leader. From the junction, stay left and continue 0.1 mile up two final switchbacks to the summit of Mount Baden-Powell (9.6 miles, 9,399'; GPS N34° 21.511' W117° 45.879'). From here, you'll have exquisite views east toward Mount Baldy above the East Fork San Gabriel River, south over the Los Angeles Basin (as far as Catalina Island on a clear day), north over the

Mojave Desert, and west over the San Gabriel Mountains, where you will soon travel. This marks the end of your long climb from the desert. You can find unsheltered camping with breathtaking views on the ridge just south of the summit.

Return to the trail junction and turn west on the PCT. The next leg of this trip stays on or near the crest and is mostly downhill and unusually straight, so you'll cover territory quickly. At each saddle between here and Throop Peak, you'll find room for one to three tents. On a clear, calm evening, these are unbeatable camping sites with the city lights far below. The trail circles the north side of Mount Burnham (8,997'), named for Lord Baden-Powell's friend and mentor who helped found the Scouting movement. On the northeast side of the mountain, at 11.1 miles, you'll find a sheltered campsite large enough for a troop of Scouts (GPS N34° 21.576' W117° 47.034').

At 12.2 miles pass the signed Dawson Saddle Trail leading down to the saddle, where you could bail out in case of bad weather. Shortly beyond is an unsigned use trail to Throop Peak (9,138'; GPS N34° 21.029' W117° 47.950'), named for Amos Throop. He founded Throop University in Pasadena, which eventually became the California Institute of Technology.

Next up is Mount Hawkins (8,850'), accessed by a 0.1-mile climbers' trail. At 13.7 miles pass the signed Hawkins Ridge Trail leading 0.4 mile to Middle Hawkins (8,505'); then enter a zone burned in the 2002 Curve Fire. At 14.7 miles is a large campsite sheltered at the edge of the burn zone.

Descend to Windy Gap at 15.1 miles. This aptly named saddle is the lowest point in this part of the San Gabriel Mountains, and it funnels masses of air moving between the desert and Los Angeles basins. Several trails radiate from the gap. Peak baggers could follow the 1.1-mile trail up to Mount Islip (8,250'), but this trip stays on the PCT. At 15.3 miles, a signed trail on the right leads down to Little Jimmy Spring (GPS N34° 20.726' W117° 49.773'). This reliable spring near two huge incense cedars is surrounded by wildflowers and has log benches where you can rest your legs for a bit. A trail continues from the spring and promptly rejoins the PCT, which reaches Little Jimmy Campground at 15.5 miles. This excellent campground has many large sites with picnic tables and stone fireplaces. If the sites near the trail are crowded or noisy, walk farther back to find some more-secluded, elevated sites. The camp and spring are named for the *Little Jimmy* comic strip, which ran in Hearst newspapers from 1904 to 1958. The cartoonist, Jimmy Swinnerton, spent summers drawing here from 1890 to 1910.

The PCT descends to Islip Saddle at 17.6 miles, where you'll cross the Angeles Crest Highway to reach another busy parking area and outhouse (GPS N34° 21.421' W117° 51.089'). Here you leave the PCT and descend the lightly used South Fork Trail (see Hike 62). Pass seasonal Reed Spring in a mile and continue down through a mix of alpine and desert vegetation to the mouth of the canyon at South Fork Campground. A grove of junipers, cypress, and non-native pines shades the sites. Walk through the campground back to your vehicle at 23 miles.

VARIATION This hike can be extended on the PCT and Burkhart Trail to become a gorgeous 41-mile backpacking trip with 10,000 feet of elevation gain. Instead of descending the South Fork Trail from Islip Saddle, follow the PCT over the shoulder of Mount Williamson. Cross the Angeles Crest Highway and follow the PCT along dramatic Kratka Ridge to Eagles Roost Picnic Area. The next section of the PCT down Little Rock Creek to the Burkhart Trail was closed at the time of this writing, so you may have to walk the highway until you can descend to Buckhorn Campground, then take the Buckhorn Trail down to the PCT near Cooper Canyon Falls and briefly jog east to meet the Burkhart Trail. You can camp and likely find water at Buckhorn Campground or Cooper Canyon Trail Camp nearby. In either case, take the Burkhart Trail over Burkhart Saddle and down to seasonal Cruthers Creek at the desert's edge. Join the Punchbowl Trail and hike above the dramatic Punchbowl past Devils Chair. Cross seasonal Holcomb Creek, where you'll find another great campsite before climbing over a last saddle and descending to the trailhead where you began.

▪ Hike 65 SMITH MOUNTAIN 🥾 🐕

HIKE LENGTH 7 miles out-and-back; 1,800' elevation gain
DIFFICULTY Moderate
SEASON October–June
MAP Tom Harrison *Angeles High Country*
PERMIT N/A

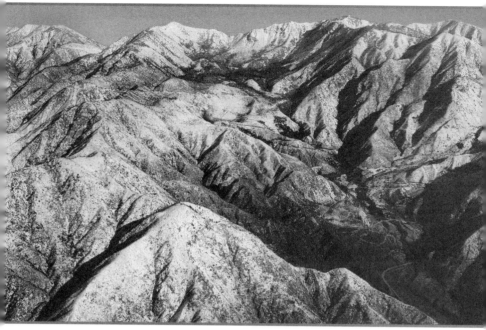

Smith Mountain is the highest peak in the left foreground. The Bobcat Fire burned everything west (left) of the Smith Mountain ridge.

■ FEATURES

Note: This hike is within the Bobcat Fire Closure Area and is closed at least through April 1, 2022. Check with the U.S. Forest Service (fs.usda.gov /angeles) before visiting.

At 5,111 feet, Smith Mountain stands tall on the divide separating the North Fork San Gabriel River from Bear Creek, smack on the eastern boundary of the rugged San Gabriel Wilderness. From its summit, you get a bird's-eye view over the eastern half of the primitive area, with the deep chasm of Bear Creek right below you. Looming close on the northwest skyline are the rocky battlements of Twin Peaks Ridge, one of the last citadels of bighorn sheep in this range.

Historians debate which Smith is the namesake of the mountain. Will Thrall argues for Eslies Smith, a Pasadena businessman who miraculously recovered from tuberculosis after staying a year at nearby Coldbrook Camp. John Robinson nominates Bogus Smith, a miner who worked the San Gabriel Canyon.

The climb is mostly by trail, but the last 800-foot rise is a steep ridge scramble, partly through brush, to the summit. Wear lug-soled boots, and do this hike when the weather is cool or cloudy; there is little shade en route.

■ DESCRIPTION

From the 210 Freeway in Azusa, take Exit 40 north for Azusa Avenue (Highway 39). Go north on Azusa Avenue, which becomes San Gabriel Canyon Road, and continue 17 miles to the Bear Creek Trail parking area, on the left at mile marker 39 LA 32.14 (GPS N34° 17.247' W117° 50.561').

Walk 2.9 miles up the well-graded Bear Creek Trail to Smith Saddle at the top of the ridge. From the saddle, leave the trail and scramble left (south) directly up the ridge, following traces of a path beaten by climbers. In some spots you must squeeze past light brush. The ridge forms the west edge of the 2020 Bobcat Fire. After taking in the superb view from the summit at 3.3 miles (GPS N34° 16.872' W117° 51.819'), return the same way. Watch your footing on the ridge descent.

■ Hike 66 BEAR CREEK ↗ 🐐 🚶 🚶

HIKE LENGTH 11 miles one-way; 1,100' elevation gain, 2,800' elevation loss
DIFFICULTY Strenuous
SEASON October–June
MAP Tom Harrison *Angeles High Country*
PERMIT Post Adventure Pass at West Fork Trailhead.

■ FEATURES

Note: This hike is within the Bobcat Fire Closure Area and is closed at least through April 1, 2022. Most of the route west of Smith Saddle burned severely. Check with the Forest Service (fs.usda.gov/angeles) before visiting.

There are no trails through the San Gabriel Wilderness. There are only trails that touch its outer perimeter and gingerly probe a short distance into its primitive sanctuary. The heart of this wilderness remains as wild as ever. The footpath that penetrates the farthest is the Bear Creek Trail into the southeastern corner of the region.

For experienced hikers who don't mind bushwhacking and boulder-hopping, this canyon jaunt is well worth the effort. A delightful stream dances and cascades under tall stands of big-cone Douglas-firs, alders, and

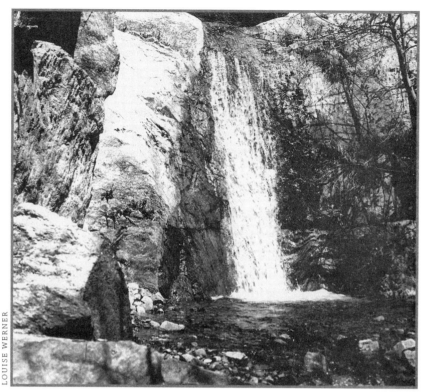

LOUISE WERNER

Falls on Bear Creek, deep in the San Gabriel Wilderness

oaks, interspaced with open chaparral glades. There are grassy flats where the canyon widens and rock-ribbed corridors where it narrows. Most of all, there is a feel of wildness. Nature reigns here; humans are the intruders. Be aware that there are many, many stream crossings; you *will* get wet, and it is unwise to attempt this hike during times of high water or just after heavy rain.

This was once grizzly bear country. In the late 1800s, hunters came in and shot them by the dozen. Pasadena historian Hiram Reid told of one such incident, which resulted in the name for the canyon: "In 1891 or '92 two or three hunters camped in the upper part of this canyon. One night a bear was caught by the hind foot in a heavy steel trap which they had set. He gnawed off his own leg and hobbled away on the bleeding stump, leaving his foot in the trap. The hunters soon discovered this in the morning, and following the bear's trail, shot him. They nailed the entrapped foot up on a tree at their camp, and I saw it there about two years later. From this incident that portion of the West San Gabriel has ever since been called 'Bear Canyon.'" Don't get this canyon confused with the Bear Canyon by Mount Baldy Village (Hike 93) or the Bear Creek by Arroyo Seco (Hike 29).

Wildflowers can be outstanding in a wet spring. I observed more than 25 species one April. I also saw a deer, four Mallard ducks, many swallowtail butterflies, many California tree frogs, two turtles, two water snakes, and an angry rattlesnake along the pristine creek. The canyon descent is particularly challenging during high water.

Today there are three wilderness campsites along the lower creek, spaced about a mile apart on shady streamside benches. These were once trail camps with stoves and fire rings, but they were so badly vandalized that the U.S. Forest Service removed all the facilities. However, they still make good overnight campsites. The trip can be done in a leisurely fashion, staying the night at one of the wilderness camps, or it can be done strenuously in one long day. Wear lug-soled boots for the many stream crossings and the stretches of boulder-hopping where the trail fades out.

Beware of ticks, rattlesnakes, poison oak, stinging nettle, and blackberry brambles along the brushy path.

■ DESCRIPTION

This trip requires a 5-mile car or uphill bicycle shuttle. From the 210 Freeway in Azusa, take Exit 40 for Azusa Avenue (Highway 39). Drive north on Azusa Avenue, which becomes San Gabriel Canyon Road. In 12 miles, you cross the West Fork San Gabriel River bridge; the spacious West Fork trailhead/staging area lies to the left, at mile marker 39 LA 27.19 (GPS N34° 14.469' W117° 52.108'). Leave one vehicle here, then continue north on Highway 39 another 5 miles to the start of the Bear Creek Trail at the edge of a large roadside turnout at mile marker 39 LA 32.14 (GPS N34° 17.247' W117° 50.901').

Wide and easy at first, the Bear Creek Trail twists and turns up through sun-struck chaparral, gaining 1,000 feet in a moderately easy 3 miles. The 4,290-foot Smith Saddle at the top of the grade marks the high point of the hike as well as the wilderness boundary. Down the other side, you descend quickly on a narrower and rougher trail, and all vestiges of civilization (save an occasional passing aircraft) instantly disappear. Tall, nearly impenetrable chaparral on the steep north slopes keeps most of the sunlight away during the fall and winter months. Young men in the Civilian Conservation Corps hacked out this trail during the Great Depression, and persistent labor has been required ever since to prevent the chaparral from reclaiming the path. To the northwest, the Twin Peaks ridge soars impressively over the far wall of Bear Creek Canyon. Caution is in order in a couple of spots where the lightly maintained trail crosses perpetually eroding ravines.

You arrive at Bear Creek's east bank at 5.6 miles. (A spectacular narrow section of Bear Creek Canyon, with vertical granite walls, begins 0.3 mile upstream from this point—worth a look if you have time for the side trip.) The small campsite here is currently overgrown, but you can find decent camping on a rise above the west bank 0.2 mile downstream (GPS N34° 16.887' W117° 53.133').

Little hint of any trail can be found in the next 4 miles as you follow the stream to its confluence with the West Fork San Gabriel River. Narrow and vegetation-choked at first, the canyon becomes wider, flatter, and talus-filled as you press on ahead. Once the stream has room to meander across the canyon floor, it curves from wall to wall, forcing you to plunge into the streamside alders and boulder-hop or wade across the water. You'll repeat that process about 25 times.

After a long, demanding canyon descent, you'll find two small campsites near a massive coast live oak on the east bank at 8.3 miles (GPS N34° 15.590' W117° 53.160'). Beyond here, conditions become somewhat easier. You'll find excellent large campsites on the west bank beside the remains of a stone cabin at 8.9 miles (GPS N34° 15.204' W117° 52.982') and at 9.3 miles (N34° 14.935' W117° 53.067').

Below the lower campsite, a well-beaten but intermittent path helps improve your speed for the last mile or so. At 10 miles you cross the West Fork San Gabriel River and join the paved West Fork National Recreation Trail, which is the main access road to Cogswell Reservoir and doubles as a bike-and-hike trail. Turn left and walk a mile out to Highway 39 and your vehicle.

VARIATION For a flat, family-friendly backpacking trip, try a 4-mile out-and-back trip from the West Fork trailhead to one of the two Lower Bear Creek campsites.

■ Hike 67 LEWIS FALLS 🡕 🐕 👫

HIKE LENGTH 1 mile out-and-back; 300' elevation gain
DIFFICULTY Easy
SEASON All year
MAP Tom Harrison *Angeles High Country*
PERMIT N/A

■ FEATURES

Green, woodsy Soldier Creek is a place of sylvan enchantment. Tucked away under high ridges in the upper reaches of the San Gabriel's North Fork, the creek seldom suffers the full glare of sunlight. Its singing waters glide and tumble beneath overarching oaks, sycamores, and alders. In summer, when the surrounding country is hot and dry, the little canyon of Soldier Creek is a damp and verdant oasis.

The trail is short—only 0.5 mile from the highway crossing to Lewis Falls (named for the late district ranger Anselmo Lewis)—but it makes up in delightful quality what it lacks in length. It is a place to saunter, rest, and contemplate; you will return from it feeling refreshed and revitalized.

■ DESCRIPTION

From the 210 Freeway in Azusa, take Exit 40 for Azusa Avenue (Highway 39). Go north on Azusa Avenue, which becomes San Gabriel Canyon Road, for a total of 20 miles. Use the roadside mileage markers to identify the starting point—a small, shaded turnout on the right at mile 34.8, where Soldier Creek tumbles through a culvert under the highway (GPS N34° 18.078' W117° 50.295').

Follow the unmarked trail up the right (east) side of the creek, passing a few privately leased summer cabins. The 2002 Curve Fire wiped out many of the historic cabins in the drainage. The trail fades out beyond the last cabin, about 0.3 mile from the highway. Scramble over boulders, crossing and recrossing the creek about 200 yards to the small clearing at the bottom of 50-foot-high Lewis Falls (GPS N34° 18.347' W117° 50.167'). Return the same way.

OPPOSITE: *Lewis Falls is a short jaunt with plenty of obstacles that are fun for the kids.*

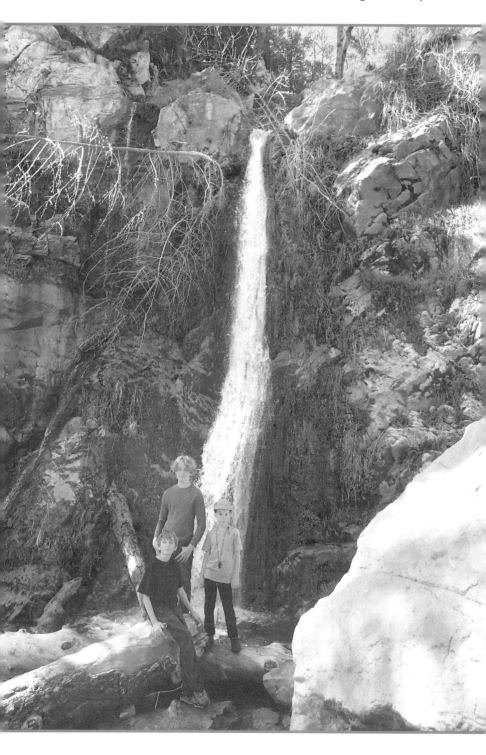

■ Hike 68 MOUNT ISLIP VIA WINDY GAP Ω 🐕 🧍

HIKE LENGTH 7-mile loop; 2,500' elevation gain
DIFFICULTY Moderate
SEASON June–October
MAP Tom Harrison *Angeles High Country*
PERMIT N/A

■ FEATURES

Note: This hike is within the Bobcat Fire Closure Area and is closed at least through April 1, 2022. Patches of forest along the route burned. Check with the U.S. Forest Service (fs.usda.gov/angeles) before visiting.

Mount Islip (pronounced "eye-slip") rises in relative isolation at the west end of the middle high country. From its 8,250-foot summit, ridges descend south to separate Crystal Lake basin from Bear Canyon, west down to Islip Saddle, and east to Windy Gap and the high country beyond. Because its cone-shaped summit stands apart from the other peaks of the mountain backbone, hikers are rewarded with an unusually fine panorama over the heart of the San Gabriels.

The mountain was named for George Islip, an early mountain pioneer who homesteaded in San Gabriel Canyon during the 1880s. In 1909 students from Occidental College, who had a summer cabin at Pine Flats (the old name for Crystal Lake basin), built a huge rock-and-wood cairn with the name Occidental on top. For many years, this Occidental Monument was a well-known landmark to hikers. In 1927 the U.S. Forest Service removed the old monument to make way for a fire lookout tower, which in turn was moved to South Mount Hawkins a decade later and then burned in the 2002 Curve Fire. Today a dilapidated old stone cabin just below the summit remains as a lone reminder of those days when searching eyes guarded the high country.

Deep in the forest, snug under the east ridge of Mount Islip, is Little Jimmy Spring. Old-timers knew this miniature, trickling watercourse as Gooseberry Spring, for the many wild gooseberry bushes that once surrounded it. It was known by this name when famed cartoonist Jim Swinnerton camped nearby in the summer of 1909. Swinnerton's *Little Jimmy* comic strip was enjoyed by Sunday-newspaper readers across the nation. Passersby that summer were often rewarded with *Little Jimmy* sketches by the camping cartoonist. Since then, the little spring and nearby campground have been known as Little Jimmy.

This is a circle trip, ascending via the old Windy Gap Trail and descending by the Islip Ridge Trail and Big Cienega Trail. Sadly, much of the once-verdant pine, cedar, and fir forest that clothed the slopes ringing the Crystal Lake basin was burned away in the 2002 Curve Fire, although scattered groves of evergreens somehow managed to survive.

■ DESCRIPTION

From the 210 Freeway in Azusa, take Exit 40 for Azusa Avenue (Highway 39). Go north on Azusa Avenue, which becomes San Gabriel Canyon Road, 24 miles to the Crystal Lake Recreation Area on the right. Drive 2.4 miles to the main hikers' parking lot at the end of the road, 0.5 mile beyond the Crystal Lake Recreation Area visitor center (GPS N34° 19.618' W117° 49.921').

Follow the signed Windy Gap Trail as it makes a gradual ascent through oaks, pines, and cedars. The trail crosses two switchbacks of the South Mount Hawkins fire road—here you begin to see the effects of the fire—and reaches a junction with the Big Cienega Trail at 1.1 miles. Go right and follow the old trail as it zigzags up the steep slope to Windy Gap at 2.4 miles. Here, you stand at one of the major trail junctions in the range. Northwest is the trail to Mount Islip; straight ahead, a portion of the Pacific Crest Trail leads to Little Jimmy Trail Camp. If you intend to spend the night, follow the latter trail, passing just above Little Jimmy Spring (purify water before drinking) before reaching the camp itself, 0.3 mile from Windy Gap. There are stoves, tables, restrooms, and plenty of little shaded flats for overnight campers.

Back at Windy Gap, follow the Islip Ridge Trail as it climbs northwest to pass another trail leading to Little Jimmy (2.6 miles) and then veers southward before gaining Mount Islip's east ridge. Our trail then continues west along the ridge a short distance to yet another junction. Turn right and follow the short pathway to the summit at 3.7 miles (GPS N34° 20.700' W117° 50.395'). Enjoy the view; it's one of the best in the range. Note the dead timber from the Curve Fire along the south-facing slopes; fortunately, the blaze failed to penetrate far past the ridgetop.

After taking in the sights, descend back down to the junction, turn right, and head southwest along Islip's south ridge to where you meet the signed Big Cienega Trail at 4.6 miles; turn left and follow it northeast and then east, through a tree graveyard, to its junction with the Windy Gap Trail at 6.3 miles. Descend the latter to the roadhead.

■ Hike 69 MOUNT ISLIP FROM ISLIP SADDLE

HIKE LENGTH 7 miles out-and-back; 1,500' elevation gain
DIFFICULTY Moderate
SEASON June–October
MAP Tom Harrison *Angeles High Country*
PERMIT Post Adventure Pass, or park outside fee area.

■ FEATURES

Note: This hike is within the Bobcat Fire Closure Area and is closed at least through April 1, 2022. Patches of forest along the route burned. Check with the U.S. Forest Service (fs.usda.gov /angeles) before visiting.

This is a scenic way to reach Little Jimmy Campground and to climb Mount Islip, starting from Islip Saddle on the Angeles Crest Highway using a section of the Pacific Crest Trail. The route has far-ranging views out over the desert and is shaded by magnificent Jeffrey and sugar pines much of the way.

■ DESCRIPTION

Exit the 210 Freeway at Angeles Crest Highway (Highway 2; Exit 20) in La Cañada Flintridge. Drive 40 miles north and east to the large Islip Saddle parking area, at mile marker 2 LA 64.0.

Little Jimmy Trail Camp
JOHN W. ROBINSON

Cross the highway and pick up the PCT leading east. Follow the well-graded trail as it climbs through chaparral and then into pines to Little Jimmy Campground at 2.0 miles (GPS N34° 20.846' W117° 49.837'). Located in a secluded little forest shallow, with stoves and restrooms, the campground is an ideal stop for overnight backpackers.

A trail near the west end of the campground switchbacks up to the east ridge at 2.6 miles, then follows the Islip Ridge Trail, as in the previous hike, to the summit (GPS N34° 20.700' W117° 50.395'). Return by the same route.

■ Hike 70 MOUNT ISLIP SOUTH RIDGE ↻ 🐕 🥾

HIKE LENGTH 10-mile loop; 2,800' elevation gain
DIFFICULTY Strenuous
SEASON May–November
MAP Tom Harrison *Angeles High Country*
PERMIT N/A

■ FEATURES

Note: This hike is within the Bobcat Fire Closure Area and is closed at least through April 1, 2022. Patches of forest along the route burned. Check with the U.S. Forest Service (fs.usda.gov/angeles) before visiting.

The south ridge of Mount Islip is prominent from many directions and offers great views. The Mount Islip Ridge Trail up this ridge is the longest and most strenuous of the three trails to the summit but is well worth the effort. With the southern exposure, this trail may be unpleasant on a hot summer day but can be climbed in the edge season when much of the high country is covered in snow.

The Mount Islip Ridge Trail that ascends this ridge from Crystal Lake was constructed in 1990 by the San Gabriel Mountains Trailbuilders, fell into disrepair after the 2002 Curve Fire, and was repaired by the Trailbuilders around 2012. This volunteer group maintains many trails around Crystal Lake and elsewhere in the range.

■ DESCRIPTION

From the 210 Freeway in Azusa, take Exit 40 to go north on Azusa Avenue (Highway 39), which becomes San Gabriel Canyon Road. Continue a total of 24 miles to the Crystal Lake Recreation Area on the right. Turn right into the recreation area and drive 1.1 miles; then turn left onto Forest Road 3N09 toward Crystal Lake. In 0.2 mile park at a trailhead lot (GPS N34° 19.133' W117° 50.686').

The unmarked and easily overlooked Islip Ridge Trail starts at the south end of the parking lot. In a minute, pass a prominent wooden sign that would have more logically been located at the start of the trail. The trail climbs to a point immediately south of Crystal Lake, which at the time of this writing has been reduced by drought to a tiny fraction of its historic size.

Switchbacks lead through the Curve Fire burn zone to gain the toe of Islip Ridge in 1.3 miles; follow the ridge upward. To the east, you have fine views of the Mount Hawkins ridge over the Crystal Lake basin. To the west, Twin Peaks and Mount Waterman are most prominent, with Mount Wilson in the distance. At about 6,700 feet, the canyon live oaks, big-cone Douglas-fir, and ponderosa pines of the lower slopes give way to Jeffrey and sugar pines that favor the cooler, higher mountainside. At this point, you may note ponderosa and Jeffrey pines growing side by side. The trees have similar stature, bark, and needles in bundles of three but can be most easily distinguished by the cones: ponderosa cones grow 3–4 inches long, while the much larger Jeffrey cones are 4–8 inches long.

At 4.0 miles reach a signed junction with the Big Cienega Trail. Continue up the ridge to a junction with the Windy Gap Trail at 4.8 miles, where you turn left and climb the last 0.2 mile to the 8,250-foot summit of Mount Islip (GPS N34° 20.700' W117° 50.395').

If the north-facing slopes are icy, you may need to return the way you came or use the Big Cienega Trail. Otherwise, you can make a loop by descending east to Windy Gap (6.0 miles). Just before the gap, you'll notice an unsigned trail on the left shortcutting to Little Jimmy Trail Camp, a great place to spend the night if you are backpacking. From Windy Gap, descend south, passing the east end of the Big Cienega Trail just before reaching the Mount Hawkins Fire Road at 7.4 miles. Take this dirt road west to the gated entrance of Deer Flats Group Campground at 8.2 miles; then continue 0.2 mile southwest on the paved campground road. At the southernmost campsites, watch for the signed Lost Ridge Trail. Take this attractive but lightly used trail south until it ends at a T-junction with the Lake Trail. Turn right and go to the upper Crystal Lake parking area; then follow the paved road 0.1 mile down to the lower lot where you began this hike.

■ Hike 71 MOUNT HAWKINS LOOP ◯ 🐕 🚶

HIKE LENGTH 13-mile loop; 3,700' elevation gain
DIFFICULTY Strenuous
SEASON June–October
MAP Tom Harrison *Angeles High Country*
PERMIT N/A

■ FEATURES

There was never a gal like Nellie Hawkins, a beautiful waitress at "Doc" Beatty's popular Squirrel Inn, high up the North Fork of San Gabriel Canyon where Coldbrook Campground lies today. From 1901 to about 1907, Miss Hawkins charmed and attracted miners, hunters, and campers—just about every mountain man for miles around. Nellie is long gone now, and the doors of Squirrel Inn have been closed for many decades, but the popular waitress will never be forgotten. Her name is eternally transfixed on two summits above Crystal Lake basin, and two other high points along the same ridge

Crystal Lake Basin. Windy Gap is the low point on the skyline, with Mount Hawkins to the right and Mount Islip to the left.

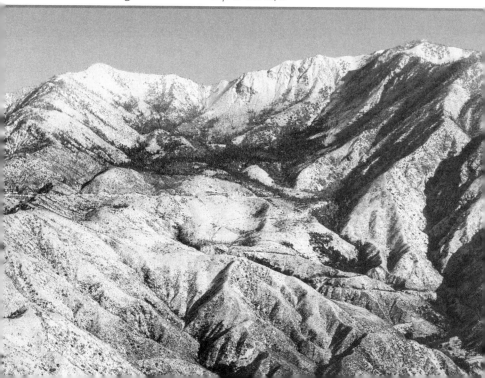

honor her informally. The two officially named peaks are Mount Hawkins and South Mount Hawkins; the two bumps on the ridge between are known to hikers as Middle Hawkins and, facetiously, Sadie Hawkins.

This circle trip climbs over or around all four of Nellie's namesakes in covering the high country northeast and east of Crystal Lake. The highlight of the trip is following the trail, built by Charles Jones and the San Gabriel Mountains Trailbuilders in the 1990s, along the ridge between Mount Hawkins and South Hawkins Lookout, with spectacular views both ways—into the Crystal Lake basin to the west and across the wild, trailless Iron Fork country to the east. Except for the short scramble up Mount Hawkins, the trip is all on trail or fire road.

The Curve Fire of September 2002 devastated the slopes around South Mount Hawkins and destroyed the historic South Hawkins Lookout Tower. The chaparral has fully recovered, but the ghostly downed timber reminds us of the inferno.

■ DESCRIPTION

From the 210 Freeway in Azusa, take Exit 40 to go north on Azusa Avenue (Highway 39), which becomes San Gabriel Canyon Road. Continue a total of 24 miles to the Crystal Lake Recreation Area on the right. Drive in 2.4 miles to the main hikers' parking lot at the end of the road, 0.5 mile beyond the Crystal Lake Recreation Area visitor center (GPS N34° 19.618' W117° 49.921').

The Windy Gap Trailhead is marked by a metal sign across the road from the parking area. The trail makes a gradual ascent through oaks, pines, and incense cedars, crosses two switchbacks of the South Mount Hawkins Fire Road, and reaches a junction with the Big Cienega Trail. Go right and follow the old trail as it zigzags up the steep slope to Windy Gap at 2.4 miles.

At the gap, turn right (east) and follow the Pacific Crest Trail (PCT) as it climbs steadily toward Mount Hawkins and across its northwest slope. Dispersed camping is possible from here to South Hawkins. The easiest route to the summit lies along the northeast spur, so you are better off to stay on the trail just past the peak and then double back and up along a climbers' trail (4.5 miles; GPS N34° 20.472' W117° 48.338').

Return to the PCT and backtrack west to the junction with the Hawkins Trail (GPS N34° 20.409' W117° 48.792'). Turn left (south) and follow the trail down the ridge, around the intervening bumps known to hikers as

Middle Hawkins and Sadie Hawkins, until you meet the fire road. Follow the latter 0.3 mile up to the site of South Hawkins Lookout tower at 8.7 miles (GPS N34° 18.698' W117° 48.628').

Descend the road down the burned west slope to the Windy Gap Trail and then back to the trailhead where you began.

■ **Hike 72 THROOP PEAK** 🥾 🐕 🚶

HIKE LENGTH 4 miles out-and-back; 1,200' elevation gain
DIFFICULTY Moderate
SEASON June–October
MAP Tom Harrison *Angeles High Country*
PERMIT N/A

■ **FEATURES**

Note: This hike is within the Bobcat Fire Closure Area and is closed at least through April 1, 2022, though it appears the trail was not damaged. Check with the U.S. Forest Service (fs.usda.gov/angeles) before visiting.

Commemorative plaque atop Throop Peak

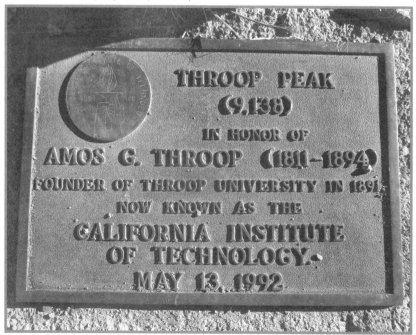

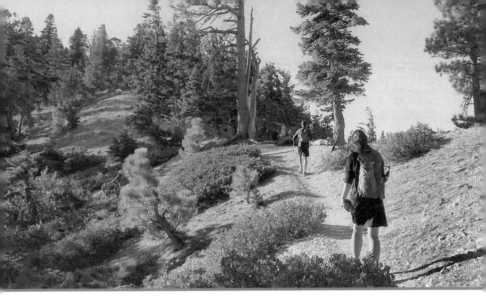

North Ridge of Throop Peak from Dawson Saddle

The Angeles Crest Highway winds through the heart of the San Gabriels like an elongated snake, reaching its highest point at the 7,901-foot Dawson Saddle. From this saddle, a prominent ridge ascends southward, reaching the crest at Throop Peak (9,138')—pronounced "troop" but named for Amos G. Throop (1811–1894), founder of California Institute of Technology.

The Dawson Saddle Trail climbs this ridge and then contours around the north slope of Throop Peak to a junction with the Pacific Crest Trail (PCT) just east of the summit ridge. It passes through an open forest of sugar and Jeffrey pines; white firs; and, higher up, lodgepole and limber pines. Most of the route offers views of the north high country and the desert far below. This is one of the best short hikes in the San Gabriel high country. Do it on a warm summer or early-fall day, when panoramas are far-reaching and the crisp high-mountain air is refreshing and invigorating.

■ DESCRIPTION

Exit the 210 Freeway at Angeles Crest Highway (Highway 2; Exit 20) in La Cañada Flintridge. Drive 45 miles north and east to Dawson Saddle at mile marker 2 LA 69.6 (GPS N34° 22.057' W117° 48.068'). If you are coming from the east, it will be faster to take Highway 138 to the Angeles Crest Highway at Wrightwood. From either direction, note that the section of CA 2 between Islip Saddle and Vincent Gap is normally not plowed in winter and is closed until April or May; check with the U.S. Forest Service or roads.dot.ca.gov to see if it's open.

The old Dawson Saddle Trail switchbacks up the ridge directly across the highway from the Dawson Saddle parking area. The new route, built by Boy Scouts in 1982 to commemorate the 75th anniversary of Scouting, begins about 150 yards down the highway to the east. Take either trail; they join atop the ridge in 0.3 mile. You walk through an open forest, first atop the ridge and then along the east slope, gently climbing southward. At 1.5 miles, where the trail bends left as the ridge of Throop rises more steeply, you can step right off the trail into a shallow bowl with a clearing sufficient for a large Boy Scout troop to camp (bring your own water).

Stay on the Dawson Saddle Trail, passing some limber pines that are found only in the San Gabriels between here and Mount Baden-Powell. At 1.8 miles, reach a signed junction with the PCT. Turn right and go about 50 yards, then veer right onto an unsigned climbers' trail. Follow this path to the summit—it's steep but easygoing (GPS N34° 21.029' W117° 47.950'). Descend the way you came.

VARIATIONS You have a choice of alternative routes on the return. You can explore the old but well-trod route that drops, steeply at first, down the northwest ridge, joining the new trail at the aforementioned bowl in 0.4 mile. Other options, requiring car or bike shuttles, are to follow the PCT east to Mount Baden-Powell and down to Vincent Gap (8 miles from Dawson Saddle to Vincent Gap; see next hike), or to go west on the PCT down to Windy Gap, Little Jimmy Campground, and Islip Saddle (also 8 miles from Dawson Saddle to Islip Saddle, see Hike 69).

■ Hike 73 MOUNT BADEN-POWELL FROM VINCENT GAP ✗ 🐕 🥾

HIKE LENGTH 8 miles out-and-back; 2,800' elevation gain
DIFFICULTY Moderate
SEASON June–October
MAP Tom Harrison *Angeles High Country*
PERMIT Post Adventure Pass, or park outside fee area.

■ FEATURES

Next to Old Baldy, Mount Baden-Powell (9,399') is probably the most popular mountain climb in the San Gabriels. A superb trail climbs directly up the northeast ridge to the summit in 40 switchbacks (the most of any trail in the range), with panoramic views north over the Mojave Desert and southeast into the deep chasm of the East Fork San Gabriel River. The trip is a living demonstration of how the forest changes with altitude: from oaks and Jeffrey pines, through white firs, into lodgepole pines, and finally a scattering of ancient, gnarled limber pines clinging to bare slopes above 9,000 feet.

For many years, the peak was known as North Baldy. In 1931 the U.S. Forest Service and U.S. Board on Geographic Names sanctioned a request by Western Regional Boy Scout Director C. J. Carlson to rename the peak after Lord Robert Stevenson Smyth Baden-Powell (1847–1941), a British Army officer who founded the Boy Scout movement in 1907. The official dedication of the new name took place on May 30, 1931, when a large party of Los Angeles–area Boy Scouts erected a plaque and flagpole on the summit. Three years later, Civilian Conservation Corps workers constructed the present 4-mile zigzagging trail from Vincent Gap to the top.

For the next 26 years, the peak was all but forgotten by the Scouts; the plaque disappeared, and the flagstaff became bent and rusted. This sad situation was brought to the attention of Michael H. "Wally" Waldron, a member of the executive board of the Boy Scouts of America, Los Angeles Area Council. Under Waldron's inspiration, more than 2,000 Boy Scouts took part in a nine-week project to erect a permanent bronze-and-cement monument on the summit. The official rededication took place on September 28, 1957. Since then, Boy Scouts have made an

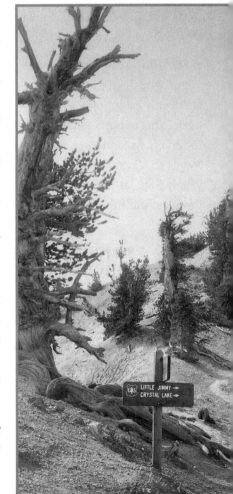

Limber pines on Mount Baden-Powell
JOHN W. ROBINSON

annual Silver Moccasin pilgrimage across the San Gabriels to the peak. On the summit ridge is a grove of weather-bent limber pines as much as 2,000 years old, identified by Angeles National Forest Supervisor Sim Jarvi in 1962. One of the largest specimens is named the Waldron Tree, in honor of the volunteer Scout leader.

■ DESCRIPTION

From I-15 north of San Bernardino, exit at Highway 138 (Exit 131) and turn west. Drive 8.6 miles to Angeles Crest Highway (CA 2), and turn left. Continue through Wrightwood and Big Pines; stay on Angeles Crest Highway for 14 miles until you reach the large trailhead parking lot at Vincent Gap at mile marker 2 LA 74.88 (GPS N34° 22.394' W117° 45.141'). Caltrans attempts to keep the highway open from Wrightwood to Vincent Gap even in the winter, but check conditions at roads.dot.ca.gov before heading this way after a storm.

A large wooden sign indicates BADEN-POWELL TRAIL—4 MILES via the Pacific Crest Trail (PCT). The trail starts up wooden steps and then switchbacks upward through a lush forest of oaks and Jeffrey pines (long needles in bundles of three; softball-size cones), with a scattering of sugar pines (short needles in bundles of five; footlong cones) and incense cedars (flat scales rather than needles) also dotting the slopes. It continues climbing steadily up the long northeast ridge of the mountain. At 1.7 miles, near the 15th switchback, a signed side trail leads left (southeast) 200 yards to Lamel Spring, which has the only water en route (unreliable in dry summers). At about 2 miles, white firs (single needles in rows rather than bundles; cones on the top of the tree that usually disintegrate before falling to the ground) begin to predominate, and shortly beyond that, the first lodgepole pines appear (thin, flaky bark; short needles in bundles of two; golf ball-size cones). As the trail tops 8,000 feet, the view opens out to the north, where the tawny expanse of the Mojave Desert fades into distant desert ranges. Now the forest thins and becomes almost exclusively lodgepole pines, tall and erect. The trail steepens, and the switchbacks shorten.

At 3.5 miles (9,000') you encounter the first aged, gnarled limber pines (short needles in bundles of five on flexible twigs; 3- to 6-inch cones resembling small sugar pine cones). The trail abruptly emerges atop the ridge, with spectacular views eastward into the Prairie Fork and the gray bulk of Old

Baldy on the skyline. Just before the final climb to the summit, the PCT branches off to the right at a junction by a 1,500-year-old gnarled limber pine called the Waldron Tree. After two more switchbacks, past scattered limber pines and lodgepole pines, the trail reaches the 9,399-foot summit, with its Boy Scout monument (GPS N34° 21.511' W117° 45.879'). The panorama is well worth the climb (providing that the lower atmosphere is not clogged with brown murkiness): a vast expanse of mountain, desert, and lowland scenery. Return the same way.

If you want to spend a night in the high country, you can find clearings to pitch a tent just south of the summit of Baden-Powell, or along the PCT above Lamel Spring.

VARIATIONS With a car or bicycle shuttle, you could continue west on this glorious section of the PCT before descending to Dawson Saddle (8 miles total; see previous hike) or Islip Saddle (12 miles total; see Hikes 64 and 69). Peak baggers have the option of visiting Mount Burnham (8,977'), Throop Peak (9,138'), Mount Hawkins (8,850'), and Mount Islip (8,250') with short detours from the PCT. If you leave a bicycle at Dawson Saddle, it's all downhill back to Vincent Gap. You'll find good camping and reliable water at Little Jimmy Campground. There's also enough space for a large party to camp just off the trail below Mount Burnham, and again a mile beyond Mount Hawkins, and many places along the ridge suitable for a single tent where you could savor million-dollar nighttime views over the Los Angeles Basin on a calm summer night.

■ Hike 74 SILVER MOCCASIN TRAIL ↗ 🐕 🚶

HIKE LENGTH 52 miles one-way; 14,600' elevation gain, 10,200' elevation loss
DIFFICULTY Strenuous
SEASON May–November
MAP Tom Harrison *Angeles High Country* and *Angeles Front Country*
PERMIT Post Adventure Pass at both trailheads, or park outside fee areas.

■ FEATURES

Note: This hike is partially within the Bobcat Fire Closure Area and is closed at least through April 1, 2022. Portions of the route between Chantry and Charlton Flats burned severely. Patches of the forest along the Angeles Crest also burned, particularly between Cloudburst Summit and Windy Gap. Check with the U.S. Forest Service (fs.usda.gov/angeles) before visiting.

The Silver Moccasin National Recreation Trail (11W06) runs the length of the San Gabriel Mountains through many of its most memorable parts. Starting through chaparral and woods and past a waterfall in Big Santa Anita Canyon, it visits the secluded West Fork San Gabriel River, Chilao's peaceful forest, Cooper Canyon Falls, and the Angeles Crest, culminating on the summit of Mount Baden-Powell. The trail was named by the Boy Scouts and is a rite of passage for thousands of boys seeking the coveted 50 Miler or Silver Moccasin badge, but the path was used for centuries by Native Americans and Anglo settlers for hunting and trade before becoming formalized in the 1930s. The trail coincides with the Gabrielino Trail from Chantry Flats to West Fork Trail Camp, with the PCT from Three Points to Vincent Gap, and with the Angeles Crest 100 ultramarathon route. The trip is long enough for you to adapt to the rhythm of trail life and lose track of time and civilization. You won't find a better trip of this length in Southern California.

There is no good group camping between West Fork and Chilao or between Cooper Canyon and Little Jimmy, so you'll face some strenuous hiking days even if you allocate a week for the trip. In the winter and spring, the ridge near Mount Baden-Powell is icy and requires an ice ax and crampons and suitable experience; unprepared hikers have died here. By late spring, water can be unreliable for 34 miles between West Fork and Little Jimmy. Check with the U.S. Forest Service (fs.usda.gov/angeles) before your trip, and cache water jugs near the Angeles Crest Highway crossings if necessary (but be sure to carry out the jugs when you collect them). You can find information about water at Cooper Canyon, Buckhorn Campground, and Lamel Spring in the Pacific Crest Trail Water Report at pctwater.com (click "Part Two, Idyllwild to Agua Dulce"). The PCT is indefinitely closed between the Buckhorn Trail and Eagles Roost to protect the endangered yellow-legged mountain frog, so this trip involves a potentially dangerous walk along the shoulder of the Angeles Crest Highway to bypass the closure. Be careful of poison oak along the trail.

The PCT segment from Vincent Gap to Three Points is closed to mountain bikers, but the Silver Moccasin segment from Three Points to West Fork is considered one of the best rides in the range for advanced cyclists.

■ DESCRIPTION

This hike begins at Chantry Flat and ends at Vincent Gap on the Angeles Crest. The 75-mile shuttle between the trailheads takes about 1.5 hours without traffic. To leave a vehicle at Vincent Gap, take I-15 to Highway 138 (Exit 131) and turn west toward Palmdale/Wrightwood. Drive 8.6 miles to the Angeles Crest Highway (CA 2), and turn left. Continue through Wrightwood and Big Pines, staying on the Angeles Crest Highway for 14 miles until you reach the large trailhead parking lot at Vincent Gap at mile marker 2 LA 74.88 (GPS N34° 22.394' W117° 45.141'). *Note:* Caltrans attempts to keep the highway open from Wrightwood to Vincent Gap even in the winter, but check conditions at roads.dot.ca.gov before heading this way after a storm. To reach the starting point at Chantry Flat, return to I-15, and take it south 15 miles to the 210 Freeway. Go west 32 miles to Exit 32 for Santa Anita Avenue in Arcadia. Drive north 5 miles to the parking lots at Chantry Flat (GPS N34° 11.734' W118° 01.347'), passing a vehicle gate that's open 6 a.m.–8 p.m. The lot fills early on weekends, so you may have to backtrack and park along the shoulder (or better yet, get someone to drop you off here.)

From the Chantry Flat Trailhead, start down the Gabrielino Trail, which begins as a gated paved road descending into Big Santa Anita Canyon. The pavement ends at 0.6 mile as you bridge Winter Creek and hike up alder-lined Big Santa Anita Canyon on a roadbed that passes some cabins and soon narrows to a foot trail.

At 1.4 miles come to a four-way junction in a tranquil oak woodland. The right branch goes to Sturtevant Falls, which is a worthy 0.3-mile detour if the creek is flowing well but generally not impressive in the summer. The left branch is recommended for equestrians or hikers who dislike heights. The middle branch is the most scenic, traversing the face above the waterfall and then following the fern-lined creek past cascades and pools. The left and middle trails reconverge at 2.2 miles.

Continuing 0.5 mile up the canyon, reach Cascade Picnic Area, where you'll find picnic tables and restrooms near the stream. You'll see many check dams built from concrete blocks resembling Lincoln logs. These dams were installed in the 1960s by the U.S. Forest Service and the Los Angeles County Flood Control District to reduce the flow of rock and sand into the Big Santa Anita Reservoir. It is hard to imagine that a road once ran through here to bring cement mixers and cranes up the canyon, or that forest managers once believed that pouring cement on a pristine creekbed was a good idea. There's something in nature that doesn't love a dam, and floods and vegetation are gradually restoring the canyon to its original character.

At 3.3 miles reach Spruce Grove Trail Camp, which has water seasonally. (*Spruce* is an older name for the big-cone Douglas-firs that thrive on this side of Mount Wilson.) At 3.5 miles the signed Sturtevant Trail veers left to reach Sturtevant Camp in 0.1 mile. This historic camp was established in 1893 and now has four cabins that you could rent with advance reservations at sturtevantcamp.com. In a pinch, you could also get water there. However, we stay on the Gabrielino Trail, which steepens as it climbs through chaparral to Newcomb Pass at 5.7 miles.

Switchback down the north side of the pass, crossing the often-closed Rincon–Red Box jeep road, to Devore Trail Camp on the West Fork San Gabriel River at 7.1 miles (GPS N34° 14.597' W118° 02.149'). Follow the trail west (upstream) to West Fork Trail Camp at 8.2 miles. Both of these fine camps have a remote feel as well as reliable water from the river—this may be the last dependable water for a long time. The Gabrielino Trail continues west, but you'll stay on the Silver Moccasin Trail, which veers north into Shortcut Canyon and then climbs to Shortcut Saddle at mile marker 2 LA 43.30 on the Angeles Crest Highway (CA 2) at 11.8 miles.

Descend to cross seasonal Big Tujunga Creek at 12.8 miles; then begin a hot climb through chaparral. At 14.5 miles pull over a low saddle to cross a service road by a picnic table. At 14.7 miles cross another paved road near the Charlton Flats picnic grounds. The trail curves around the hillside, passing a spur to Vetter Mountain at 15.3 miles; it then meets paved Forest Road 3N16B in the picnic grounds at 15.5 miles. Hike north through a gate; then leave the road at a hairpin turn and continue north along the East Fork of Alder Creek. Eventually, the trail climbs out to meet Forest Road 3N21 near the Chilao Campground Little Pines Loop, just north of the Angeles Crest Highway at 17.6 miles (mile marker 2 LA 49.69). The first-come, first-served campground sometimes has piped water.

Continue on the Silver Moccasin Trail through a pine forest, over a low ridge, and down to the edge of Upper Chilao Picnic Area at 18.2 miles, where you might again find a working faucet. At 18.6 miles recross FR 3N21 at the Chilao Trailhead. Pass Horse Flats Campground (no water) at 19.7 miles, and then the Bandido Group Camp (also no water) at 20.1 miles. The trail now turns east and parallels the paved Santa Clara Divide Road to its junction with the Angeles Crest Highway at Three Points (mile marker 2 LA 52.85), where you'll find trailhead parking and an outhouse at 22.2 miles.

The rest of your route coincides with the PCT. Climb near the Angeles Crest Highway, crossing it three times to reach Cloudburst Summit at 27.0 miles by mile marker 2 LA 57.04 (GPS N34° 21.088' W117° 56.063'). Follow the circuitous trail down (or take a shortcut down the dirt service road) into Cooper Canyon to find a spacious and scenic trail camp shaded by pines at 29.7 miles. Seasonal water flows in the nearby creek. At 31.0 miles reach a junction with the Buckhorn Trail. Cooper Canyon Falls is just to the east and is well worth a visit if the creek is flowing. The PCT is closed ahead indefinitely to protect the habitat of the endangered yellow-legged mountain frog. Unless the closure has been lifted, our route turns right and climbs the Burkhart Trail, passing two waterfalls, to reach Buckhorn Campground at 32.6 miles. You may find working water spigots at the campground.

Walk up through the campground and find the paved exit road leading east to meet the Angeles Crest Highway at mile 2 LA 59.05 at 33.4 miles. You now face a dull and dangerous walk along the shoulder of the highway to Eagles Roost picnic area at 36.1 miles (mile marker 2 LA 61.65). (If the endangered species detour has been lifted, you could get here by walking 3.3 miles along the PCT from the Buckhorn Trail junction.)

The PCT resumes along Kratka Ridge with stunning views, then crosses back to the north side of the highway at 37 miles (mile marker 2 LA 62.50). It then climbs high onto the shoulder of Mount Williamson, passes a spur leading to Williamson's summit, and drops back to cross the highway once more at Islip Saddle at 39.9 miles (mile marker 2 LA 64.0).

Beyond the saddle, begin a long, gradual climb toward Mount Baden-Powell. Watch for red currants, which ripen by late summer. At 42.2 miles you'll reach the spacious Little Jimmy Trail Camp, named for cartoonist Jimmy Swinnerton, who drew the *Little Jimmy* comic strip and spent his summers here from 1890 to 1910. The historic camp has picnic benches and stone ovens. If the campsites near the trail are full or noisy, look farther back for more-private spots. Less than a quarter mile beyond the camp, you'll find reliable Little Jimmy Spring beside two huge incense cedars and many wildflowers.

Staying on the PCT, reach aptly named Windy Gap at 42.5 miles (GPS N34° 20.602' W117° 49.720'). Pressure differences between the desert and valley air masses funnel air through this low point in the Angeles Crest. A web of trails radiates from the gap; be sure to continue east on the PCT. At 42.9 miles pass an undeveloped large campsite at the edge of the burn zone from the 2002 Curve Fire. Continue past climbers' trails leading to Middle Hawkins, Mount Hawkins, and Throop Peak to reach a signed junction with the Dawson Saddle Trail at 45.5 miles.

The next section of the trail, along the Angeles Crest, is perhaps the best part of the whole trip. You'll find a small exposed tent site with amazing views here, and at each saddle between Throop and Baden-Powell. At 46.6 miles bypass Mount Burnham on the north side. You'll find another campsite large enough for a troop of Scouts on the northwest slope of the mountain. Major Fredrick Burnham was a cofounder of the Boy Scout movement. At 47.9 miles reach a short trail on the right leading to the 9,399-foot summit of Mount Baden-Powell. A monument here celebrates Lord Robert Baden-Powell (1857–1941), who founded the Boy Scouts in 1907. You can find more-exposed camping on the ridge south of the peak. The only trees growing this high are lodgepole and limber pines, which favor the tallest mountains in Southern California. Lodgepole pines have needles in bundles of two and round, golf ball–size cones, while limber pines have needles in bundles of five and longer, 4- to 6-inch cones on their flexible branches. The Wally Waldron Tree at the junction below the summit is a twisted limber pine believed to be 1,500 years old.

The trip concludes with 40 knee-jarring switchbacks descending to Vincent Gap. Halfway down, you'll pass three undeveloped campsites and then a signed spur at a switchback that leads 100 yards to seasonal Lamel Spring, in a ravine.

■ Hike 75 BIG HORN MINE ↗ 🐐 ⚙

HIKE LENGTH 4 miles out-and-back; 500' elevation gain
DIFFICULTY Easy
SEASON June–October
MAP Tom Harrison *Angeles High Country*
PERMIT Post Adventure Pass, or park outside fee area.

■ FEATURES

Gold mining—both placer and lode—has played a long and prominent part in the saga of human beings in the San Gabriels. One of the most famous of the lode mines was the Big Horn, perched at 6,900 feet on the rocky east slopes of Mount Baden-Powell. Its weather-battered, crumbling remains are among the most photogenic reminders of the once-feverish mining era in the mountains.

From Vincent Gap, a wide trail (the remains of an old wagon road) contours around the massive east flank of Baden-Powell to the mine ruins. The route, shaded by stands of Jeffrey pines and white firs, offers an almost continuous panorama down into the East Fork San Gabriel, with Baldy and its sister peaks rising as a massive backdrop. This is an ideal trip for both the history buff and the photographer.

It was mountain man Charles "Tom" Vincent, a fugitive whose real name was Charles Vincent Daugherty, who discovered the Big Horn in 1894—the climax of a multiyear search for the lode that fed the rich placers of the East Fork. Vincent, a prospector and hunter who lived from about 1870 until 1926 in a crude log cabin high in Vincent Gulch, sold the mine to a group of investors, who spent a fortune to develop it. Thousands of feet of tunnels were bored, and heavy equipment was laboriously hauled in. For slightly more than a decade, the Big Horn prospered. The California Division of Mines reported a yield of nearly $40,000 in gold from 1904 to 1906. But, as with all San Gabriel mining ventures, the veins petered out and the effort was abandoned. The property was finally acquired by the U.S. Forest Service in 2007 to become part of the Sheep Mountain Wilderness.

■ DESCRIPTION

From I-15 north of San Bernardino, exit at Highway 138 (Exit 131) and turn west toward Palmdale/Wrightwood. Drive 8.6 miles to the Angeles Crest

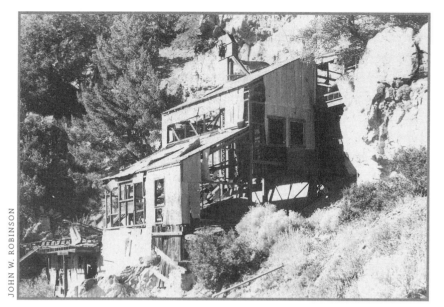

Big Horn Mine stamp mill

Highway (CA 2), and turn left. Continue through Wrightwood and Big Pines, staying on the Angeles Crest Highway for 14 miles until you reach the large trailhead parking lot at Vincent Gap at mile marker 2 LA 74.88 (GPS N34° 22.394' W117° 45.141'). *Note:* Caltrans attempts to keep the highway open from Wrightwood to Vincent Gap even in the winter, but check conditions at roads.dot.ca.gov before heading this way after a storm.

The trail, distinctive but unmarked, leaves the Vincent Gap parking area, drops about 60 feet, and begins to contour southeast around the mountain. Much of our hike is shaded by tall Jeffrey pines and white firs, with an occasional sugar pine rising above the others. In 0.2 mile, stay right at a signed junction where the Mine Gulch Trail drops into the canyon. In another 0.5 mile, pass above Vincent's well-preserved cabin, hidden in the woods (GPS N34° 22.075' W117° 44.664').

Watch for a small mine tunnel, the beginning of the Big Horn complex. As you round the massive buttress of Mount Baden-Powell, the deep gorge of the East Fork of the San Gabriel River, and its tributary canyons come into full view; the grayish mass of Old Baldy looms beyond. The trail rises about 300 feet to top a ridge and passes the foundations of mine buildings. As you round a bend, the old stamp mill comes suddenly into view, clinging to the precipitous, rocky hillside (GPS N34° 21.405' W117° 44.664'). This is Big Horn Mine, and here the broad trail ends. The main tunnel is just behind and above the mill building; it extends several hundred feet into the mountain, is usually wet, and is unsafe to explore beyond the entrance. An old footpath, narrow and partly overgrown, continues about 0.5 mile farther around the mountain, passing several small prospects. The big mill building is dilapidated and dangerous to enter, as a NO TRESPASSING sign indicates. But don't be disappointed; the views from trail's end of the huge mill, as well as views out over the gorge of the East Fork to Old Baldy, are well worth the trip.

VARIATION It is possible to climb the east ridge of Mount Baden-Powell from where the Big Horn Mine wagon road rounds the bend just east of the mine. This steep ridge climbs 2,400 feet over 1.5 miles and is suitable only for adventurous hikers comfortable with cross-country travel. Loop back on the Pacific Crest Trail for a memorable 8-mile hike.

■ Hike 76 UPPER EAST FORK 🥾 🐐 🧍

HIKE LENGTH 8 miles out-and-back; 2,000' elevation gain
DIFFICULTY Moderate
SEASON May–October
MAP Tom Harrison *Angeles High Country*
PERMIT Post Adventure Pass, or park outside fee area.

■ FEATURES

This scenic hike is the best way to reach the upper East Fork country. You leave the Angeles Crest Highway at Vincent Gap and descend the broad, sloping V of Vincent Gulch 4 miles to the great bend, where the East Fork's main channel elbows east and becomes Prairie Fork. This trip is a favorite of anglers; some fine trout swim in this cold mountain stream. Remember that this is an "upside-down" hike—all uphill on the return.

The upper East Fork country is rich in history as well as scenic attractions. Charles "Tom" Vincent—mountain man, prospector, and hunter of bighorn sheep, grizzly bears, and deer—settled here sometime before 1880. His rustic cabin, high up in Vincent Gulch, was filled with the horns and skulls of game he had shot. Prairie Fork was so named because early settlers herded cattle there to feed on the rich grasses. It is said that two perpetrators

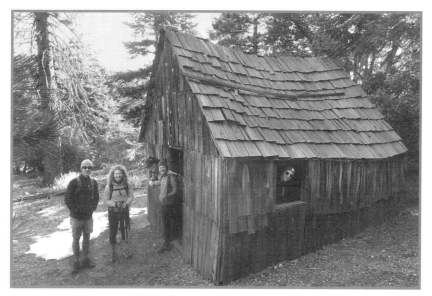

Tom Vincent's cabin still stands high above the East Fork. Treat it with care so others can enjoy.

of the 1857 Mormon Massacre in Utah built the first cabin in Prairie Fork, settling there to hide from the law. During the early 20th century, gold was recovered from the rock walls of Prairie Fork at the Native Son Mine. The mine's six tunnels have been idle since the early 1920s.

■ DESCRIPTION

From I-15 north of San Bernardino, exit at Highway 138 (Exit 131) and turn west toward Palmdale/Wrightwood. Drive 8.6 miles to the Angeles Crest Highway (CA 2), and turn left. Continue through Wrightwood and Big Pines, staying on the Angeles Crest Highway for 14 miles until you reach the large trailhead parking lot at Vincent Gap at mile marker 2 LA 74.88 (GPS N34° 22.394' W117° 45.141'). *Note:* Caltrans attempts to keep the highway open from Wrightwood to Vincent Gap even in the winter, but check conditions at roads.dot.ca.gov before heading this way after a storm.

From Vincent Gap, walk south on the closed wagon road toward Big Horn Mine. In 0.2 mile, turn left at a signed junction onto the Mine Gulch Trail, which actually descends Vincent Gulch. Soon, watch for a faint spur to Vincent's cabin. The trail stays on the right (west) slope for a while, and then crosses the small creek and parallels it close to the east bank for most of the remaining distance down. The trail may be confusing as it starts to bottom out at 3 miles; be sure to stay in the main canyon and not stray into one of the canyons to the east. However, you can find an excellent sheltered campsite about 100 yards up the second canyon on the east after reaching the bottom of Vincent Gulch (GPS N34° 21.356' W117° 43.591').

At 4.1 miles, reach a prominent confluence with Prairie Fork on the left (GPS N34° 20.612' W117° 43.475'). Watch for the wreck of a Schweitzer 2-32 glider that departed the Llano gliderport and got trapped on this side of the ridge in 1974.

A trail once led up Prairie Fork to Cabin Flat Campground and beyond, but this canyon burned and is now a nasty bushwhack through stinging nettles, poison oak, and wild rose brambles. You can find a flat, gravelly area to camp in the main wash near the confluence with Prairie Fork.

Return the way you came.

East Fork San Gabriel River

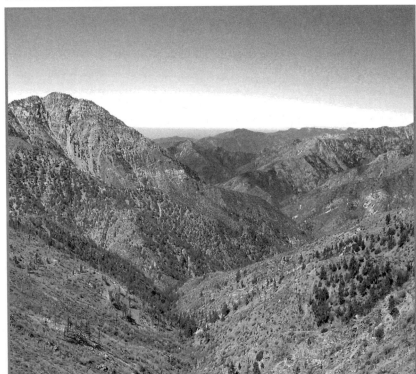

DOUG CHRISTIANSEN

■ Hike 77 BRIDGE TO NOWHERE 🥾 🐕 🥾

HIKE LENGTH 10 miles out-and-back; 800' elevation gain
DIFFICULTY Moderate
SEASON November–June
MAP Tom Harrison *Angeles High Country*
PERMIT Post Adventure Pass. Get free self-issued wilderness permit at trailhead.

■ FEATURES

The saga of the East Fork San Gabriel can just about be summed up in one word: *gold*. The precious metal was discovered in the canyon gravels in 1854, and almost overnight the East Fork became a scene of frenzied activity. Eldoradoville, the only real gold rush town in the San Gabriels, sprang up where the East Fork elbows north. It boasted three hotels and a half dozen saloons. Not much more is known about Eldoradoville, for the rustic boomtown was washed away lock, stock, and barrel in the great flood of 1862. Placer gold was exhausted soon thereafter, and prospectors began searching nearby

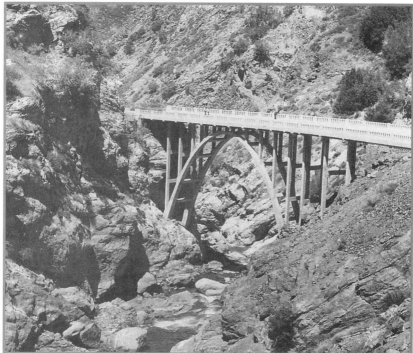

JOHN W. ROBINSON

Bridge to Nowhere in the Narrows of the East Fork

draws and hillsides for promising quartz veins. Their efforts were rewarded, and for the next half century, lode gold was recovered from tunnels and shafts along canyon sides and well up on higher slopes. Place names in the area today commemorate the miners of yesteryear—Heaton Flat, Trogden's, Allison Gulch, and Shoemaker Canyon, to name a few.

The East Fork is quiet now, save for the rush of the stream and the rustling of oak and alder leaves. Prospectors still pan for gold but no longer burrow for hidden treasures. The scars of the gold-mining efforts can be seen on almost the entire length of the chasm. You must look up along canyon slopes to see these aged marks; all evidence of streamside mining activities has long since been erased by the torrential floods that periodically scour the streambed.

Los Angeles County developed an ambitious plan to cut a road up the East Fork San Gabriel River all the way to Blue Ridge and down to Wrightwood. Prison work crews got as far as the mouth of the Narrows and constructed a massive concrete bridge across the gorge before another great flood in 1938 washed away their efforts, leaving the "Bridge to Nowhere" stranded miles beyond the remaining roadhead.

This is an interesting trip for more than historical reasons. The scenery here is monumental, on a scale seen nowhere else in the San Gabriels. The gorge of the East Fork cuts deep into the eastern high country, separating such giants of the range as Mount Baden-Powell and Old Baldy. The rise from the floor of The Narrows (2,800') to the top of Iron Mountain (8,007') is 5,200 feet in 1.75 horizontal miles! This is nature in its grandest proportions (at least by Southern California standards). You can find dispersed camping on benches above the East Fork, and there is good trout fishing in the broad stream.

A word of warning: Do not attempt this trip after heavy rains. There are numerous stream crossings en route, and storms turn this usually bubbling creek into a raging torrent that is dangerous, if not impossible, to ford.

■ DESCRIPTION

From the 210 Freeway in Azusa, take Exit 40 north for Azusa Avenue (Highway 39), and follow Azusa Avenue into San Gabriel Canyon. In 11.9 miles, turn right (east) on East Fork Road. At a hairpin turn in 5.3 miles, stay straight (east) on a minor road that crosses a bridge and ends in 0.9 mile at a parking lot and closed gate (GPS N34° 14.227' W117° 45.917'). Get a free self-issued wilderness permit at a box near the entrance to the lot.

Walk north along the roadbed that follows the high bench east of the river for 0.5 mile before dropping to the canyon floor. Your trail now follows the river, fording its shallow but rushing waters 14 times. You pass remnants of the old East Fork Road, which was destroyed by the flood. At 2.7 miles you pass under Swan Rock, a towering wall west of the river with the outline of a giant swan etched in gray. When the canyon broadens and curves northwest, climb to your right and follow the old roadbed high above the river. You then cross 50 acres of private property and reach a massive highway bridge seemingly out of place. This is the famous Bridge to Nowhere, the most imposing remnant of the East Fork Road of yesteryear (GPS N34° 17.001' W117° 44.803').

Most hikers turn around here. But if you continue upstream another 0.25 mile, you will reach a pool in the river near the mouth of the Narrows, where you can escape the crowds and frolic in the water. On your return, watch for bighorn sheep, especially just south of the bridge.

VARIATION If you have time and energy, consider a visit to Devil Gulch Falls. Walk back under the bridge and follow the river south half a mile, rounding a bend to the mouth of the first canyon on the west, Devil Gulch. Hike up this rough canyon for 200 yards, passing the foundation and chimney of a miner's cabin, to the splendid but well-hidden waterfall (GPS N34° 16.826' W117° 45.276'). Continue south along the rough bank of the river to rejoin the main trail in a mile.

■ Hike 78 UP THE EAST FORK ↗ 🐕 🚶

HIKE LENGTH 16 miles one-way; 4,500' elevation gain
DIFFICULTY Strenuous
SEASON November–June
MAP Tom Harrison *Angeles High Country*
PERMIT Post Adventure Pass. Get free self-issued wilderness permit at trailhead.

■ FEATURES

This long canyon trip—best savored as an overnight backpack—traverses the middle and upper sections of the East Fork, from the lower ranger station to the junction of Vincent Gulch and Prairie Fork, and then ascends the former to the Angeles Crest Highway at Vincent Gap. En route, you pass through some spectacular canyon scenery and visit historic mining

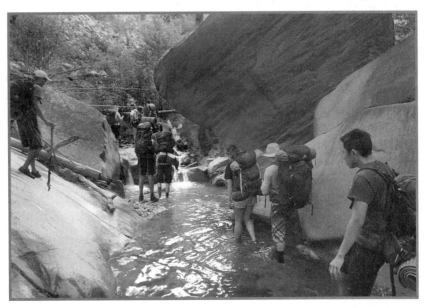

Wading up the East Fork Narrows

areas—most notably Heaton Flat, where Billy Heaton settled and mined in the 1890s; Iron Fork, once the home, vegetable garden, and social meeting place of miner George Trogden; and Mine Gulch, the lair of hunter/miner/ mountain man Charles "Tom" Vincent. The mines are gone, but there are some inviting wilderness campsites in the upper canyon.

This trip can be done in one long day if you're in a hurry, but it's much more enjoyable to stay the night in the canyon, sleeping in primitive wilderness campsites alongside the stream under stately live oaks. A long car shuttle is required between the East Fork Trailhead and Vincent Gap. As an alternative, making the trip easier, you can reverse the trip and go downstream instead of up. The trip should not be done when the water is high; there are dozens of stream crossings en route.

The old Pacific Light & Power (PL&P) Trail, built in 1911 for access to a planned power plant, clings to the cliffs high on the west side of the Narrows. Segments can still be seen, but it is no longer continuously passable. Several mines can also be found on the slopes above the Narrows.

■ DESCRIPTION

This trip requires a 1.5-hour, 81-mile car shuttle. Leave a getaway vehicle at Vincent Gap Trailhead. From I-15 north of San Bernardino, take Exit 131 for Highway 138. Take Highway 138 west 8.6 miles, then turn left onto the Angeles Crest Highway (CA 2); continue 14 miles to the Vincent Gap Trailhead parking lot at mile marker 74.88 (GPS N34° 22.394' W117° 45.141'). Drive your other vehicle to the East Fork Trailhead. Return to I-15 and go west on the 210 Freeway about 24 miles to Azusa. Take Exit 40 north on San Gabriel Canyon Road (Highway 39) and drive 12 miles to East Fork Road, where you turn right. Continue up East Fork Road 6 miles to a parking lot at the end (GPS N34° 14.227' W117° 45.917'). You can get a self-issued wilderness permit at a box by the outhouse. Better yet, have a friend drop you off and then pick you up later (caution: there is no cell coverage at East Fork).

From the East Fork (lower end), proceed 5 miles upcanyon to The Narrows, as described in the previous hike, to a good spot for a snack break beside the river at the mouth of the Narrows just above the bridge. If you watch carefully, you'll find at least 10 primitive campsites between here and Mine Gulch. Your travel now becomes much slower through The Narrows to the Iron Fork junction at 6.6 miles, where you can find primitive camping at the site of Trogden's former cabin. It is generally easier to walk near the river, fording as necessary, rather than fight through the alder thickets. Continuing through the interesting and sometimes challenging canyon, and

Descending the East Fork

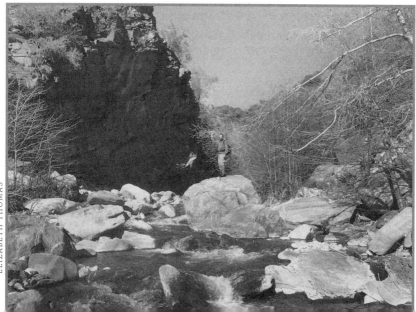

ELIZABETH THOMAS

passing a thin waterfall at the lip of Falls Gulch, you'll find a splendid wilderness campsite opposite the confluence with Fish Fork at 8 miles (GPS N34° 18.334' W117° 43.953').

Above Fish Fork, the canyon becomes less precipitous. Follow the river to Mine Gulch at 11.8 miles, where three tributaries—Mine Gulch, Vincent Gulch, and Prairie Fork—join to form the main East Fork. You could find a gravelly clearing among the boulders to camp here just below the Prairie Fork junction. Watch for the wreckage of a Schweitzer glider from 1974. Soon pick up the trail up Vincent Gulch to Vincent Gap.

■ Hike 79 RATTLESNAKE PEAK ⟳ 🐕

HIKE LENGTH 9.5-mile loop; 4,000' elevation gain
DIFFICULTY Strenuous
SEASON October–April
MAP Tom Harrison *Angeles High Country*
PERMIT N/A

■ FEATURES

Rattlesnake Peak (5,862') is the second-most inaccessible major summit in the San Gabriels, after Iron Mountain. A steep climbers' trail ascends the south ridge from Shoemaker Canyon Road and descends the east ridge. The

Rattlesnake Peak in the springtime is a great place to find horned lizards. Their camouflage is so effective that you rarely see them unless they are moving.

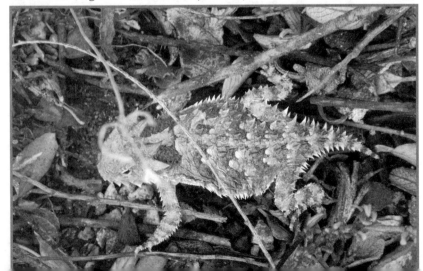

difficulty varies depending on how recently hikers and wildfires have beaten back the chaparral. The 2012 Williams Fire burned 4,192 acres, including most of Rattlesnake Peak; at the time of this writing, the brush has regrown but is not too bad along the route, and visitors have cut it back in places.

The U.S. Forest Service does not track information about this route, so your best bet is to search online for recent trip reports to make sure that other hikers are getting through before you venture up here. Long pants, long sleeves, boots with good tread, trekking poles, and gaiters will all be helpful. Go on a cool day. Rattlesnakes are no more common here than elsewhere at this altitude, but lizards are plentiful.

■ DESCRIPTION

From the 210 Freeway in Azusa, take Exit 40 for Azusa Avenue (Highway 39), and follow it north into San Gabriel Canyon. In 11.9 miles turn right on East Fork Road. Go 3.4 miles; then bear left on the paved Shoemaker Canyon Road (Forest Road 2N11) at mile marker 3.39. Continue 1.9 miles to a vehicle gate and parking area (GPS N34° 14.060' W117° 46.244').

From the gate, hike up the so-called Road to Nowhere for 1.5 miles. Watch for mile markers placed by the overly optimistic roadbuilders. Just before a gully at mile marker 3.39 (GPS N34° 14.962' W117° 45.887'), turn left off the road up a steep trail. You'll soon find yourself on traces of another abandoned road cut. At 1.7 miles leave the cut at a saddle and follow a climbers' trail steeply up the ridge, going west, then northwest, and then west again. Chamise, scrub oak, and buckwheat dominate the vegetation. Several ridges intersect at a bump just above 4,000 feet (2.5 miles; GPS N34° 15.127' W117° 46.557'). Note this point carefully in case you need to retrace your path. Our ridge, rocky in places and steep in others, turns north and continues past some false summits to Rattlesnake Peak, 4.2 miles from the start (GPS N34° 16.310' W117° 46.620'). The summit benchmark is named Fang. Enjoy outstanding views in all directions, especially northeast toward Iron Mountain and Baldy.

You can return the way you came, but if the brush is not too bad, it is more fun to descend the east ridge. Carefully stay on the crest of the ridge, disregarding occasional animal paths that drop down the side, and quickly enter thick chaparral. Below 4,600 feet, the ridge steepens, and at times you can boot-ski down the sandy parts. This is much better for descent than for climbing. At 3,650 feet (5.8 miles; GPS N34° 15.909′ W117° 45.287′), the climbers' trail abruptly turns right off the ridge and makes steep switchbacks southward. At 3,050 feet, you join a good path contouring along the abandoned road cut (GPS N34° 15.763′ W117° 45.476′). You soon reach the mouth of the northern tunnel and join the Shoemaker Canyon Road at 6.8 miles. From here, it's easy walking through a second tunnel back to the trailhead.

■ Hike 80 IRON MOUNTAIN ⤢ 🐕

HIKE LENGTH 14 miles out-and-back; 6,200′ elevation gain
DIFFICULTY Strenuous
SEASON March–June
MAP Tom Harrison *Angeles High Country*
PERMIT Post Adventure Pass. Get free self-issued wilderness permit at trailhead.

■ FEATURES

At 8,007 feet, Iron Mountain is by far the least accessible peak in the San Gabriels. It towers as a mighty sentinel at the west end of San Antonio Ridge, standing perpetual guard over the East Fork San Gabriel River, whose waters rampage a mile below. No formal trails approach its isolated summit, and to climb it you must start miles away and thousands of feet below.

East Fork miners knew it as Sheep Mountain, for the large herds of bighorn sheep that once made their home on its rugged flanks. Today Iron Mountain is a last citadel of these "statuesque masters of the arid crags," as author and zoologist A. Starker Leopold described them. Easily disturbed by man, about 400 bighorn sheep remain in the most isolated recesses of the range.

This is a long, extremely strenuous climb for the first 2,500 feet on trail, and the last 3,500 feet up is a narrow climbers' path on a chaparral- and forest-covered ridge. Do it only if you are in excellent physical condition. Wear lug-soled boots and carry two full water bottles. This trip can be dangerous under wintry conditions, when the ridge becomes icy. Someone signing the summit register called this "the mother of all hikes," and it certainly is the single most strenuous mountain in this book.

■ DESCRIPTION

From the 210 Freeway in Azusa, take Exit 40 north for Azusa Avenue (Highway 39). Follow Azusa Avenue into San Gabriel Canyon. In 11.9 miles, turn

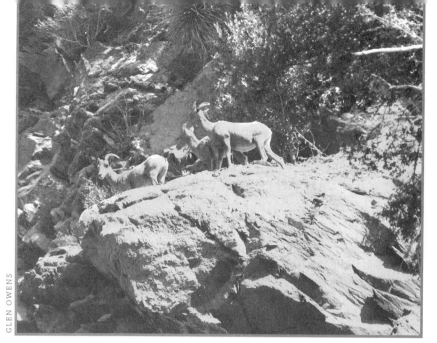

Nelson bighorn sheep in East Fork

right (east) on East Fork Road. At a hairpin turn in 5.3 miles, stay straight (east) on a minor road that crosses a bridge and ends in 0.9 mile at a parking lot and closed gate (GPS N34° 14.227' W117° 45.917'). Get a free self-issued wilderness permit at a box near the entrance to the lot.

Walk north 0.5 mile along the fire road, above the East Fork and around two bends, to the beginning of the Heaton Flat Trail. Turn right and follow the signed Heaton Flat Trail east to the ridgetop, and then northeast along the ridge to 4,582-foot Allison Saddle, 4.3 miles from the start, where the maintained trail ends. Climb north, directly up the ridge, following a distinct path worn in by climbers over the years. You reach a small saddle at 6,100 feet. Above it, you're climbing in a forest of pines and firs, a great improvement over the thorny chaparral. Continue up the ridge to the forested summit, where you will find a U.S. Geological Survey benchmark and a register left by Sierra Club climbers (GPS N34° 17.304' W117° 42.801'). In the register, a scribe once wrote, "Through bad chaparral and stinging nettle; to do Big Iron you need pants of metal."

Walk a few feet in any direction to enjoy a superb panorama, one of the best in the whole range. The peak falls sharply off in every direction except east, where broken San Antonio Ridge joins Iron Mountain to the Baldy massif. Descend the way you came. The next hike describes the epic traverse to Baldy.

VARIATION Hikers have also posted trip reports of Iron Mountain ascents via the southwest ridge from Alison Gulch and the north ridge from Fish Fork. Both are extremely demanding, with inevitable bushwhacking and extensive scrambling on poor rock.

■ Hike 81 SAN ANTONIO RIDGE ↗ 🐕

HIKE LENGTH 16 miles one-way; 6,000' elevation gain, 10,200' elevation loss
DIFFICULTY Strenuous
SEASON May–November
MAP Tom Harrison *Angeles High Country*
PERMIT Post Adventure Pass and get free self-issued wilderness permit at East Fork.

■ FEATURES

Get set for a spectacular and extremely challenging traverse along the spine of the San Gabriel Mountains. From the top of Old Baldy, you descend a net elevation of 8,000 feet to East Fork San Gabriel River by way of San Antonio Ridge and Iron Mountain. Done in the manner described here (net downhill), the trip is certainly the most tortuous hike of all those included in this book. Doing it in reverse, from East Fork to Badly, is a test piece if you're a real glutton for punishment.

It's prudent to know the area well before attempting this trip. Climb Baldy (see Hike 94) and Iron Mountain (see previous hike) on their own, and be sure neither feels overly demanding. You'll want to wear boots, long pants, and gaiters. Trekking poles can be helpful for the long, steep, loose descents. Some hikers who are uncomfortable on loose Class 3 rock will find a rope helpful. If you are doing this as a day trip, you'll want 6 quarts of water on a cool day, or more in the summer. Although it is possible to camp on the summit of Baldy or Iron, or on flat spots along San Antonio Ridge, you may need to haul 10 quarts or more of water for such an arduous backpacking trip.

■ DESCRIPTION

This trip requires a 1-hour car shuttle. Leave a getaway vehicle at the East Fork Trailhead: From the 210 Freeway in Azusa, take Exit 40 north on Azusa Avenue (Highway 39), and drive 11.9 miles to East Fork Road, on the right. Continue up East Fork Road 6 miles to a parking lot at the end (GPS N34° 14.227' W117° 45.917'). You can get a self-issued wilderness permit at a box

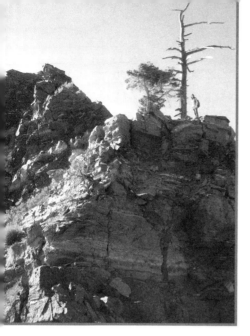

Climbing out of Gunsight Notch

by the outhouse. Return to the 210 and go east 12 miles; take Exit 52 for Base Line Road. Turn left to go west on Base Line for 0.2 mile; then turn right (north) on Padua Avenue. In 1.8 miles turn right onto Mount Baldy Road. Follow it 11.7 miles to Manker Flats, where you can park or get dropped off alongside the road (GPS N34° 15.966' W117° 37.614').

You begin with the standard approach to Old Baldy's summit from the Manker Flat Trailhead by way of the Baldy Bowl Trail (see Hike 94) at 4.0 miles (GPS N34° 17.351' W117° 38.780'). You might be tempted to take the ski lift, but check the current schedule (baldyresort.com/mountain/hours-of-operation) because it may not be running at the early hour you'll need to start this trip.

From Old Baldy's summit, proceed west to 9,988-foot West Baldy at 4.3 miles. From there you can visually trace the rounded San Antonio Ridge in the distance as it curves gradually left and finally becomes a serrated spine leading to Iron Mountain's summit. Based on what you can see, estimate how long it will take you to walk over to Iron Mountain, then multiply that figure by at least two.

From West Baldy, you descend through talus and timberline krummholz (stunted, almost prostrate trees) and then through taller trees to the first saddle in the ridge (7,772'). On the undulating ridge ahead, you travel through sparse groves of timber and thickets of snowbrush, a low-growing but thorny variety of ceanothus. The USGS topo map shows trails connecting several old mines in the upper Coldwater Canyon drainage to the south, but the mines and trails alike have been abandoned for decades.

The crux of the trip begins at Gunsight Notch, the lowest point along the ridge, at 7.7 miles (7,350'; GPS N34° 17.391' W117° 42.019'). Work your way over and around pinnacles of shattered metamorphic rock on the arête, mostly a slow process of stepping over or bashing through low chaparral. Bighorn sheep tracks may guide you. Take great care not to pull on or otherwise dislodge blocks of rock; many seem to be delicately balanced and poised to tumble. Also make sure that no two climbers are in the same fall line. While you're on this tense stretch, try to relax occasionally and enjoy the dizzying vistas into the precipitous Fish Fork canyon to the north and the gentler Coldwater Canyon drainage to the south.

When you finally reach Iron Mountain's 8,007-foot summit at 8.6 miles (GPS N34° 17.304' W117° 42.801'), you'll find a register appropriately labeled Big Bad Iron. Take a long breather on top and revel in the view. Some nice camp or picnic sites can be found amid the scattered pines just below the summit. When it's time to leave, head down the south ridge on a rather well-beaten but occasionally steep climbers' path. Huge yuccas, some with a thousand slender daggers, grow uncomfortably close to the path. Keep your speed down lest you slide into one of them. A couple of pine- and-fir dotted flat areas on the way down offer a chance to rest and cool off. At the 4,582-foot Allison Saddle (11.1 miles), you come upon the comparatively well-maintained Heaton Flat Trail, which zigzags southeast up a hill, gaining about 150 feet, then descends, more or less steadily to Heaton Flat. From there, walk out on the service road to the East Fork Trailhead.

■ Hike 82 MOUNT BALDY NORTH BACKBONE TRAVERSE ↗ 🐐 🚶

HIKE LENGTH 11 miles one-way; 5,100' elevation gain
DIFFICULTY Strenuous
SEASON June–October
MAP Tom Harrison *Angeles High Country*
PERMIT N/A

■ FEATURES

This trip traverses the San Gabriel Mountains from south to north, climbing over Mount Baldy and following its rugged North Backbone over Dawson Peak and Pine Mountain, the second- and third-highest peaks in the range after Baldy itself. The North Backbone looms high over the broad swath of the Prairie Fork, razor-sharp ridges plunging nearly vertically into dim forested

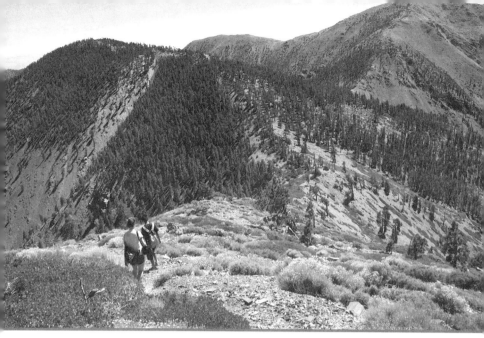

On the North Backbone between Pine and Dawson

recesses. The long drive is justified by the fantastic scenery and seclusion of Sheep Mountain Wilderness. If you bring enough water, you could spend the night on any of the summits. Beware: These north slopes hold snow and ice in the spring long after the south-face snow has completely melted.

■ DESCRIPTION

This trip requires a 75-minute car shuttle. From the I-15/Highway 138 junction at Cajon Pass, drive northwest on Highway 138 for 8.6 miles, and then west on CA 2 for 5.3 miles to Wrightwood. At mile marker 2 SBD 1.00, turn left onto Spruce Street, then immediately right onto Apple Avenue, then immediately left onto Acorn Drive. Follow Acorn Drive 0.6 mile to where it becomes a private road, and park off the pavement (GPS N34° 21.261' W117° 38.505'). Drive the other car back down to I-15 and then south to the 210 Freeway and west to Exit 54 for Mountain Avenue in Upland. Take Mountain Avenue north and stay on it as it turns right then back left (west), passes San Antonio Dam and Fire Station, and eventually reaches a T-junction with Mount Baldy Road in 4.2 miles. Turn right and drive 9 miles up to the Manker Flat trailhead parking area (GPS N34° 15.966' W117° 37.614').

Follow the Baldy Bowl Trail 4.0 miles to the summit of Mount Baldy (see Hike 94). Paths radiate in all directions from the top and can be misleading, especially in whiteout conditions. Descend the steep North Backbone Trail on the north side to a saddle of 8,800 feet; then follow the trail that climbs steeply up to 9,575-foot Dawson Peak at 5.3 miles (GPS N34° 18.185' W117° 38.158'). Dawson Peak was named for Ernest Dawson, who served as the Sierra Club Angeles Chapter outings chair from 1916 to 1927 and as president from 1935 to 1937. His son Glen was a pioneering rock climber of the Sierra Nevada, establishing the first route up the East Face of Mount Whitney in 1931.

Descend the far ridge 0.5 mile to meet a junction with the unmaintained Dawson Peak Trail, which soon fades to oblivion as it drops westward into Fish Fork Canyon. Stay north on the Backbone Trail over 9,648-foot Pine Mountain; a 100-foot detour is necessary to reach the true summit at 6.3 miles (GPS N34° 18.809' W117° 38.655'). Then drop back down the sharp ridge to a saddle shortly before reaching an unmarked trailhead on Forest Road 3N06 at 7.6 miles (GPS N34° 19.755' W117° 38.187').

Follow a use path up to the Pacific Crest Trail on the north side of the road, and continue west as it contours around Wright Mountain. At 8.6 miles, turn north onto the Acorn Trail, and follow it down to the top of Acorn Drive at 10.7 miles. Continue 0.2 mile to a gate, then another 0.4 mile down the paved private road to your vehicle.

VARIATION The North Backbone can also be hiked from Blue Ridge as a 7.5-mile out-and-back with 4,100 feet of elevation gain. From Inspiration Point on CA 2 at mile marker 2 LA 78.00, drive 7.2 miles east on Blue Ridge Road (initially signed FR 3N26, soon becoming 3N06) to a turnout above the prominent saddle between Pine and Wright Mountains. This dirt road is usually passable by low-clearance vehicles unless it has been damaged by a storm. Follow the undulating North Backbone over Pine and Dawson to Baldy, and then return the way you came.

■ Hike 83 BLUE RIDGE TRAIL 🡕 🐕 👫 ◉ 🚶

HIKE LENGTH 5 miles out-and-back; 1,300' elevation gain
DIFFICULTY Easy
SEASON June–October
MAP Tom Harrison *Angeles High Country*
PERMIT N/A. Free first-come, first-served walk-in camping.

■ **FEATURES**

This is a pleasant uphill walk on the north slope of Blue Ridge. Your trail starts up through stands of scrub oaks, black oaks, and Jeffrey pines, giving way to white firs, sugar pines, and lodgepole pines as you climb over 7,000 feet. Vistas are far-reaching—first, north over Table Mountain to the tawny desert expanse and then, atop Blue Ridge, south into the yawning chasm of the East Fork San Gabriel River, with Mount Baldy, Iron Mountain, and Mount Baden-Powell as imposing backdrops. This is a hike you should stroll rather than stride, savor rather than gulp. Go slowly and enjoy nature's delights.

■ **DESCRIPTION**

From the junction of I-15 and Highway 138, turn west and drive 8.6 miles to the Angeles Crest Highway (CA 2). Turn left and continue through Wrightwood; stay on the Angeles Crest Highway for 9 miles until you reach the Big Pines Information Station at mile marker 02 LA 80.00 (GPS N34° 22.693' W117° 41.349').

The Blue Ridge Trail starts near the restrooms opposite the information station. It briefly descends to a lower trailhead and then begins climbing south. Follow the trail as it climbs around a low ridge, drops to a trickling watercourse, and then steadily climbs through open forest. You cross a dirt road and zigzag higher, with views opening to the north, over Table Mountain to the desert. After 2.3 miles you reach the top of Blue Ridge and a junction with Forest Road 3N06 and the Pacific Crest Trail (PCT). Right across the road is Blue Ridge Campground, with tables, stoves, and restrooms. For the best view southward into the deep gorge of the East Fork, walk 0.3 mile up FR 3N06 or the PCT (GPS N34° 21.408' W117° 40.991').

You may wish to stay the night at Blue Ridge Campground before returning the way you came. Bring your own water.

■ **Hike 84 JACKSON LAKE LOOP** ○ 🐎

> **HIKE LENGTH** 7-mile loop; 1,300' elevation gain
> **DIFFICULTY** Moderate
> **SEASON** May–October
> **MAP** Tom Harrison *Angeles High Country*
> **PERMIT** Post Adventure Pass, or park outside fee area.

■ FEATURES

The oak-and-pine-forested slopes between Jackson Lake and Vincent Gap are just as lovely as the Blue Ridge above Wrightwood. In the spring, chickadees sing, and lupine, paintbrush, and wallflower lend color to the woods. Visitors are lured by a chain of fine campgrounds and picnic areas along Big Pines Highway. Jackson Lake, a natural sag pond on the San Andreas Fault, is stocked with fish and well used by anglers and picnickers. Those looking to stretch their legs will enjoy this hike, climbing up on the Jackson Lake Trail, then following the Pacific Crest Trail (PCT) and a segment of dirt road before descending the Boy Scout Trail back to the lake. The trails are in good condition but are oddly not shown on USGS or U.S. Forest Service maps.

■ DESCRIPTION

From I-15 north of San Bernardino, exit at Highway 138 and turn west. Drive 8.6 miles to Angeles Crest Highway (CA 2), and turn left. Continue through Wrightwood on Angeles Crest Highway for 9 miles; at mile marker 2 LA 80.00, turn right on Big Pines Highway (County Road N4) and proceed 3.0 miles to signed Jackson Lake, on the left. Take this road 0.2 mile to the parking lot by the lake (GPS N34° 23.538' W117° 43.682').

From the west end of the parking area, take the signed Jackson Lake Trail, which climbs steeply for 0.1 mile to a dirt Forest Service road. Turn left and follow the road, passing above a campfire circle for a youth camp. At 0.7 mile veer left at a fork. Pass the signed Boy Scout Trail on the right, by which you will return; then soon reach another sign for Jackson Lake Trail on the right at 0.8 mile (GPS N34° 23.478' W117° 43.940'). Follow this scenic trail as it climbs to meet the PCT at 2.1 miles (GPS N34° 22.920' W117° 44.492').

Turn right (west) on the PCT. Immediately pass a fork on the left leading a few yards up to Forest Road 3N26. Take the trail or road west until they rejoin. This is 0.6 mile by the road or 0.8 mile by the more scenic trail. Cyclists are prohibited on the PCT and must choose the road.

From the second junction, continue west on FR 3N26, passing a locked gate. Veer right at a hairpin turn onto the signed Boy Scout Trail at 3.7 miles (GPS N34° 23.039' W117° 45.437'). At 4.2 miles, reach the signed Fenner Saddle Trail dropping down the ridge to the north. Walking 50 yards along the ridge brings you to a bench with a pleasant view. Our hike remains on the

Boy Scout Trail back to the dirt road near where your trip began at 6.2 miles. Turn left and promptly reach the fork in the road.

You could turn right and return the way you came, but, for a change of scenery, turn left instead and continue 0.2 mile on the rough road. Watch for the unsigned Serra Trail on the right (GPS N34° 23.551' W117° 44.044'), descending a draw just beyond a sharp bend in the road. Take this trail, which eventually widens to become an abandoned dirt road. In 0.5 mile stay right at a fork in a large clearing, and soon reach the short trail down to Jackson Lake.

VARIATION For a shorter trip, turn around at the PCT and return on the Jackson Lake Trail the way you came. This option is 4.2 miles with 1,300 feet of elevation gain.

■ Hike 85 BIG DALTON MYSTIC LOOP ⟳ 🐕

HIKE LENGTH 3-mile loop; 1,300' elevation gain
DIFFICULTY Moderate
SEASON November–April
MAP Tom Harrison *Angeles High Country*
PERMIT N/A

■ FEATURES

This loop offers a great workout in a short distance by climbing hills on both sides of the mouth of Big Dalton Canyon. It is an appealing destination for a brisk morning or evening walk, especially in the springtime when the slopes are green, the creek is flowing, and the wildflowers are out. The parking area is outside of Big Dalton Canyon, so the trail is accessible even when the park is closed to vehicles. Some parts of the trail are very steep; shoes with good tread are essential, and a trekking pole might be helpful. The canyon is named for Henry Dalton, an Englishman who came to California in 1843 and established Rancho Azusa de Dalton, which became the region's second-largest landholding.

■ DESCRIPTION

From the 210 Freeway in Glendora, take Exit 44 for northbound Lone Hill Avenue. In 1.0 mile turn left on Foothill Boulevard. In 0.5 mile turn right on Valley Center Avenue. In 0.8 mile turn left on Sierra Madre then immediately right on Glendora Mountain Road. In 0.5 mile park at a turnout on the left just beyond Big Dalton Canyon Road (GPS N34° 09.386' W117° 50.206').

From the trailhead, walk back south on Glendora Mountain Road for 0.3 mile to the entrance to Linder Equestrian Park. Find the signed Wren Meacham Trail at a bridge over the Big Dalton Wash behind a brick building. Cross both channels on bridges, and then walk upstream along the wash to a sign at 0.6 mile where the trail turns right and begins climbing steeply through the sage scrub and elderberry onto the hillside south of Big Dalton Canyon. Beware of poison oak in places. Weave and climb along the wooded slope; then descend as abruptly as you climbed, reaching the creek at 1.4 miles. The trail leads upstream, crossing the creek three times, to reach the signed north end of Wren Meacham on Big Dalton Canyon Road at 1.6 miles.

Directly across the road, take the signed Mystic Trail that begins climbing steeply again up the hillside on the north wall of the canyon. At 2.3 miles pass a spur on the left that shortcuts to the Poopout Trail, but stay on Mystic to reach a flagpole at a hairpin turn on the Lower Monroe Fire Road (2N16) at 2.5 miles (GPS N34° 09.802' W117° 50.068').

From here, you could take the fire road (now deteriorated to a trail) in either direction to Glendora Mountain Road. Going left leads 2.4 miles down to the mouth of Little Dalton Canyon at mile marker 13.9, while going right climbs 5.0 miles to the ridge at a huge turnout 0.3 mile east of mile marker 5.6. Our route, however, turns hard left and follows the steep Poopout Trail directly down the ridgeline for 0.6 mile to return to your parked vehicle.

VARIATION A maze of trails laces the floor and east wall of Big Dalton Canyon. You could spend an enjoyable morning exploring these paths.

■ Hike 86 MARSHALL CANYON LOOP ⟳ 🐕 👫

HIKE LENGTH 4.5-mile loop; 800' elevation gain
DIFFICULTY Moderate
SEASON October–May
MAP Tom Harrison *Angeles High Country*
PERMIT N/A

■ FEATURES

Between the deep gorges of San Gabriel Canyon to the west and San Antonio Canyon to the east lies a region of low-lying, chaparral-coated ridges and meandering, oak-shaded canyons. The eastern San Gabriel Valley lies

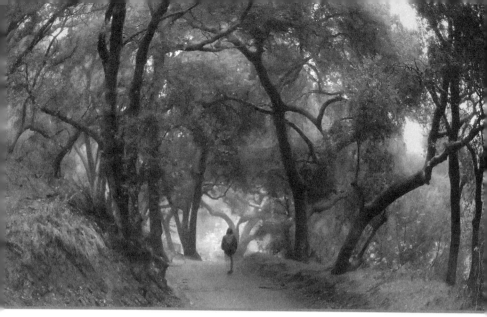

Walking beneath the oaks on a rainy morning in Marshall Canyon

immediately to the south; north is the private San Dimas Experimental Forest. Most of the foothill trails are rather short with modest elevation gains, perfect for a casual hike. It's ideal country for a stroll on a cool winter or spring afternoon, when the creeks are bubbling, the foothill grasses are a luxuriant deep green, and the hillsides are clothed in wildflowers.

Perhaps the best of these trails lies in Marshall Canyon Regional Park, just above La Verne. The trip described here is mostly on smooth, well-graded dirt road or trail and passes through a classic Southern California foothill landscape of hillsides and glens. The park is popular, especially on weekends, so you will likely find yourself sharing the trail with other hikers, mountain bikers, and equestrians (horses have the right-of-way). Although the canyon is a maze of trails and dirt roads, almost all of them eventually wind up back at the canyon entrance, so it's difficult to get truly lost. Poison oak is plentiful in the canyon, so don't stray off the trail.

■ DESCRIPTION

From the 210 Freeway in La Verne, take Exit 48 north on Fruit Street. In 0.1 mile turn left on Base Line Road. After 0.3 mile, turn right on Esperanza Drive. Follow Esperanza 2.1 miles, and then turn right on Stephens Ranch Road. Proceed 1.0 mile past a golf course to the signed Equestrian Assembly Area, a large dirt parking area on the right (GPS N34° 09.111' W117° 44.745').

From the east end of the parking lot, descend to a paved road and follow the trail along the north side of the road. The unpromising start passes a yellow gate at 0.2 mile and squeezes between a Los Angeles County Probation Department camp and a sewage treatment plant before reaching the signed Fred Palmer Equestrian Camping and Training facility at 0.4 mile. Turn left at the sign and follow a fire road as it winds generally northeast through shady oaks above the creek. At 1.1 miles, come to a three-way junction with two other trails leading to the right. Stay left on the fire road. You will make a loop that returns on the rightmost trail to this point. The middle trail is a shortcut that rejoins the fire road.

As you continue up the fire road, you will soon come to another trail on the right that parallels the fire road for 0.2 mile before rejoining; you may take either path. Soon after, the fire road starts climbing in earnest. Pass a picnic area nestled in the oak trees beside the creek at the head of the canyon. The fire road turns south and comes to another junction where a trail on the right shortcuts back to the three-way junction you passed earlier. But this hike continues east up the fire road until it reaches the gate to Claremont Hills Wilderness Park at 2.2 miles (see next hike).

Turn right to follow another broad fire road southwest, pass a set of benches, and continue until you can turn right onto another fire road at 2.6 miles that leads back to Marshall Canyon. Descend for 0.5 mile on this fire road until you reach a junction; here, take the trail right and switchback down the hill and across the creek, returning to the three-way junction at 3.4 miles. Turn left on the fire road and retrace your steps for a mile back to the parking area.

VARIATION This loop connects to a maze of other interesting trails. You can spend many pleasant visits exploring the other trails in Marshall.

For an optional one-way trip, go up Marshall Canyon and down the Claremont Hills Wilderness Park. From Baseline Road in Claremont, drive north 1.5 miles on Mills Avenue to Claremont Hills Wilderness Park (see next hike). Leave one car here, and the other at the Marshall Canyon Trailhead. Proceed up the route described above until you reach the wilderness park. Turn left or right; both routes involve a 2.5-mile, mostly shadeless descent on fire road down to the Claremont Trailhead and your car, for a total one-way distance of just under 5 miles.

■ Hike 87 CLAREMONT HILLS WILDERNESS PARK
Ω ⋔ ♟

HIKE LENGTH 5-mile loop; 900' elevation gain
DIFFICULTY Moderate
SEASON All year
MAP Tom Harrison *Angeles High Country*
PERMIT Parking fee

■ FEATURES

Claremont Hills Wilderness Park, established in 1996, has become an extremely popular loop for hiking, biking, running, and strollers, receiving an estimated 500,000 annual users. On a clear winter day, it offers views of the snowcapped summits of San Jacinto, San Gorgonio, and Ontario Peaks and out to the skyscrapers of downtown Los Angeles towering beyond countless subdivisions. On a perfect day, you can even see Catalina Island. The trail is on a good fire road that is normally well graded, but it can wash out during winter rains. The park can be unpleasantly hot on summer afternoons and is occasionally closed during times of extreme fire danger, including county red-flag warnings.

■ DESCRIPTION

From the 210 Freeway in Claremont, take Exit 52 for Base Line Road and drive west. In 0.7 mile turn right on Mills Avenue. Go up the hill 1.2 miles to the large Claremont Hills Wilderness Park trailhead parking area, on the right at the corner of Mount Baldy Road, or an even larger lot beyond at the top of Mills (GPS N34° 08.564' W117° 42.465'). The lots have a fee and often fill on busy mornings, and there is no legal street parking nearby. Be aware that the City of Claremont aggressively enforces parking restrictions here. Consider parking on Mills near Base Line and biking to the trailhead.

From the trailhead, follow the dirt road past the Thompson Creek Dam flood-control basin and across a seasonal creek. The path forks in 0.2 mile—take the right fork up Cobal Canyon, then loop around to return to this junction via Burbank Canyon. Hiking alongside Cobal Creek in the oak-shaded canyon is one of the most pleasant parts of this trip. At 1.0 mile the road leaves the canyon at a switchback and climbs unrelentingly up the ridge. At a water tank at 1.5 miles, the dirt West Fork Palmer Evey Motorway leads east toward Palmer Canyon and Potato Mountain. The Wilderness Park loop veers west and, at 2.0 miles, reaches a saddle at the northernmost point of the park.

The loop continues along an undulating ridge to the southwest. This area burned on Halloween night in 2003, leaving a scorched, barren landscape, but the sage scrub has rebounded well. Common plants include California buckwheat, laurel sumac, California sagebrush, and black sage. At 2.2 miles, pass a gate on the right at the top of the fire road leading up from Marshall Canyon (see previous hike). Soon after, you'll pass shaded benches placed on the hill by the Rotary Club in memory of Claremont mayor Nick Presecan, who helped preserve the park. At 2.5 miles, pass another fire road leading to the right down into Marshall Canyon.

Soon crest the last of the rolling hills and begin the steady descent. At 3.4 miles, you reach yet another junction to Johnson Pasture, but our trip turns hard left and descends on the switchback. Descend the brushy slopes of Burbank Canyon overlooking Thompson Creek Dam and return to the main fork where you started the loop. Turn right, cross the creek, and reach the parking lot.

■ Hike 88 ETIWANDA FALLS ↻ 👫

HIKE LENGTH 5-mile loop; 1,200' elevation gain
DIFFICULTY Moderate
SEASON All year
MAP Tom Harrison *Angeles High Country*
PERMIT N/A

■ FEATURES

One of the Inland Empire's rare accessible waterfalls is hidden near the mouth of East Etiwanda Canyon just out of sight of millions of commuters. This moderate hike to the falls follows a good dirt road all the way and loops back to explore the rest of the preserve.

The route passes through the North Etiwanda Preserve, which protects an area of diverse habitats and significant cultural history. Part of the 1,200-acre preserve was initially set aside in 1998 to offset the impact of 210 Freeway development, and the preserve formally opened in 2009. Situated on an alluvial fan between two washes and bisected by the Sierra Madre Fault, this alluvial sage scrub and fragile riparian habitat is home to 15 animal species and two plants that are endangered, threatened, or of other special concern, including the San Bernardino kangaroo rat and the southwestern willow

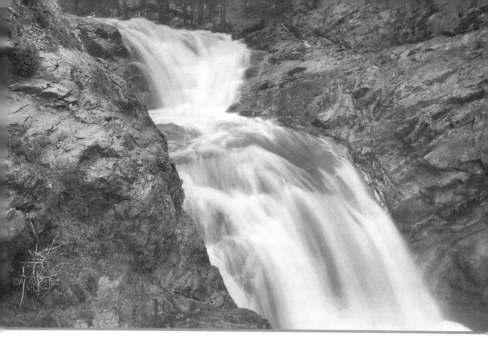

Etiwanda Falls at high flow

flycatcher. It's a great place to watch for lizards, birds, and wildflowers. *Remember that all the plants and animals in the preserve are protected.*

The area was long used by the Tongva and Serrano peoples. The Spanish established Mission San Gabriel in 1771, then granted the 13,000-acre Rancho Cucamonga to Tiburcio Tapia in 1839. George Day purchased a parcel at the mouth of the canyon in 1867 and built a ditch and then a flume for irrigation; the area is now crisscrossed with numerous historic and modern irrigation systems. This hike can be done as a 3.5-mile out-and-back to the falls, but if you have time, it's even better to loop back and see more of North Etiwanda Preserve.

■ DESCRIPTION

From the 210 Freeway just west of I-15, take Exit 61 for Day Creek Boulevard in Rancho Cucamonga. Drive north and then east 2.1 miles; then turn left onto Etiwanda Avenue and proceed 0.4 mile to the end of the road, where you'll find the trailhead parking (GPS N34° 09.935' W117° 31.398'). Pay close attention to parking restrictions—the city has aggressively towed vehicles.

From the parking area, gated dirt roads lead north and west into Etiwanda Preserve. Head north toward the mountain. The alluvial fan sage scrub community along the trail was once plentiful but is now endangered by heavy development north of the 210 Freeway and by containment of the creeks. Common species include California sagebrush and buckwheat, white sage, ceanothus, and scale broom. In 0.2 mile, pass the main kiosk on the left, where you can learn more about the preserve. At 0.6 mile, come to a four-way junction. The preserve loop turns left. If you walk 500 feet to the right, you'll come to a picnic area overlooking East Etiwanda Wash. This trip heads straight north on the unsigned road to the falls.

The path soon exits the preserve and enters the San Bernardino National Forest. At 1.1 miles, continue straight at another four-way junction. Pass another gate and continue along the flank of the deep wash. At 1.7 miles, the road ends at the top of the falls, which usually run year-round (GPS N34° 11.159' W117° 31.400'). Enjoy the overlook, but take care on the slick rock. A short use trail leads up a canyon to the left to another smaller waterfall.

You can return the way you came (3.5 miles round-trip) or make a 5-mile loop by hiking back to the northernmost four-way junction and turning west to reenter Etiwanda Preserve in a burn zone near mile marker 1.5. The May 2014 Etiwanda Fire scorched 2,190 acres after an illegal campfire got out of control. Fortunately, sage scrub is adapted to recover rapidly from wildfires. Continue counterclockwise on the preserve loop. At the highest point along the route, a spur forks right to visit a gaging station on Day Creek, but your path turns south toward a prominent scarp with two trees beside a picnic bench and restroom. From here you can enjoy magnificent views over the Inland Empire to San Gorgonio, San Jacinto, and Santiago Peaks.

Continuing on the loop, come to a boardwalk overlooking a freshwater bog. This sag pond, the vista point you just came from, and another scarp ahead are all products of the Cucamonga Fault Zone, which relieves the tremendous pressures produced as the San Gabriel Mountains have thrust upward. Your path, now a deteriorating asphalt road, drops down to meet a power-line road. Turn left (west) and soon emerge at the trailhead where you began.

■ Hike 89 STODDARD PEAK ↗ 🐴

HIKE LENGTH 6 miles out-and-back; 1,000' elevation gain
DIFFICULTY Moderate
SEASON All year
MAP Tom Harrison *Angeles High Country*
PERMIT N/A

■ FEATURES

Stoddard Peak (4,624') is located on the shoulder of Ontario Peak overlooking San Antonio Canyon. Despite its diminutive stature among the huge peaks circling the canyon, Stoddard offers excellent views of Mount Baldy and is an enjoyable exercise hike or half-day excursion. The peak and nearby canyon were named for William Stoddard, who, in 1880, founded the first of many mountain resorts in this area. These resorts were immensely popular before the development of air-conditioning. Ranchers sent their families up into the high country to escape the oppressive heat that blankets the Inland Empire during the summer months.

In 2017, The Conservation Fund acquired 230 acres around the trailhead to establish the Mt. Baldy Wilderness Preserve that protects watershed, wildlife corridors, and open space in San Antonio Canyon.

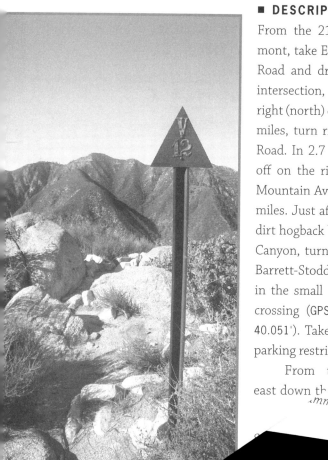

■ DESCRIPTION

From the 210 Freeway in Claremont, take Exit 52 onto Base Line Road and drive west to the first intersection, Padua Avenue. Turn right (north) onto Padua and, in 1.8 miles, turn right on Mount Baldy Road. In 2.7 miles, pass the turnoff on the right for Shinn Road/Mountain Avenue and proceed 3.7 miles. Just after you pass over the dirt hogback blocking San Antonio Canyon, turn right at the sign for Barrett-Stoddard Road and park in the small lot before the bridge crossing (GPS N34° 13.372' W117° 40.051'). Take care to obey ⸀ parking restrictions. *hike*

From the ⸀ *cross the*

east down th ⸀ *summit*

bridge over San Antonio Creek. On the west side of the creek, you can see traces of the old Mount Baldy Road that once ran along the creek before being washed out one too many times. Follow Barrett-Stoddard Road past some private residences near Barrett Canyon and, at 0.8 mile, pass a gate. Continue, generally southward, past the mouth of Cascade Canyon and above the flat-topped Spring Hill, where traces of an old farm can still be seen. At 2.5 miles, cross a saddle to reach Stoddard Flat. Look to the right (west) for a trail chopped through the chaparral (GPS N34° 12.107' W117° 39.762'). Follow it up the hill and then along the rocky crest of a ridge. Hike 0.4 mile, passing two false summits before you reach the true summit of Stoddard Peak at the south end of the ridge (GPS N34° 11.793' W117° 39.934'). Return the way you came.

VARIATION Another option is to descend 2.2 miles cross-country along Stoddard's south ridge over Peak 4,324 to a fenced viewing platform above the Lower San Antonio Fire Station on Mountain Avenue beside San Antonio Creek. The fire station is 0.3 mile off Mount Baldy Road.

■ Hike 90 SUNSET PEAK 🐾 🐐 ☀ 🥾

HIKE LENGTH 6 miles out-and-back; 1,200' elevation gain
DIFFICULTY Moderate
SEASON All year
MAP Tom Harrison *Angeles High Country*
PERMIT N/A

■ FEATURES

In winter and early spring, when snow blankets the high peaks of the range and the air is crisp and clear, the ascent of Sunset Peak is a particularly rewarding experience. From the 5,796-foot summit, you get a grandstand ꞈ sta of the great horseshoe ridge—crowned by massive Mount Baldy— de ͮircles upper San Antonio Canyon. To the northwest, beyond the Crystal of the East Fork country, looms the line of peaks above It's an effort to take in tle. Even in the summ the 3-mile fire road to the summit, well worth the panorama under winter's glistening man- excellent hike as long as you go in the morning or evening, when the trail is shaded. Consider coming for a sunset picnic or to spend the night on the top.

■ DESCRIPTION

From the 210 Freeway in Claremont, take Exit 52 for Base Line Road. Go west on Base Line for 0.2 mile, then turn right (north) on Padua Avenue. In 1.8 miles, turn right onto Mount Baldy Road. Follow it 7.1 miles to Mount Baldy Village. Just as you approach the village, turn left on Glendora Ridge Road and go 0.8 mile to Cow Canyon Saddle, where parking is available on the shoulder (GPS N34° 13.682' W117° 40.222'). Be aware of signed parking restrictions. If the gate at the bottom of Glendora Ridge Road is closed, park outside the gate and hike the road.

Proceed past the locked gate up the fire road that winds through shady big-cone Douglas-fir and chaparral up the north side of Sunset Peak. At 1.9 miles, at a junction with Forest Road 2N07, make a sharp switchback. Just after a second switchback at 2.5 miles, bear left on a firebreak and head southwest straight to the summit at 2.9 miles (GPS N34° 12.995' W117° 41.364'). This worthwhile and fun shortcut, with some easy rock scrambling at the top, saves time and distance over the alternative—a mile of tedious road walking. On top, you'll find cement pillars and a rainwater collection system from the fire lookout tower that stood here from the 1920s to the 1970s. After taking in the splendid panorama, descend the way you came.

VARIATION For a shorter but steeper climb (1.5 miles each way), you can take the steep firebreak all the way from Cow Canyon Saddle.

VARIATION Sunset Peak can also be climbed via FR 2N07, which starts at a saddle on Glendora Ridge Road at mile marker 7.78, 4.2 miles from Mount Baldy Road. This is 4 miles each way with 1,350 feet of elevation gain on a well-maintained fire road with excellent views.

VARIATION Sunset Ridge Fire Road continues all the way to San Dimas Canyon Road at mile marker 1.32, near the top of San Dimas Dam. This trip is 15 miles with 1,500 feet of elevation gain and 4,700 feet of loss. Keen-eyed hikers will notice use trails descending firebreaks from Sunset Ridge Fire Road to Evey Canyon, Claremont Hills Wilderness Park, and Marshall Canyon.

■ Hike 91 SAN ANTONIO FALLS 🡕 🐕 👫

HIKE LENGTH 1.2 miles out-and-back; 200' elevation gain
DIFFICULTY Easy
SEASON April–November
MAP Tom Harrison *Angeles High Country*
PERMIT N/A

■ FEATURES

San Antonio Creek begins as a snow-fed trickle high up on the east face of Mount Baldy. It gains strength as it descends the canyon and then cascades down a series of steep drops. The final and most impressive three-level drop is called San Antonio Falls. This short hike leads to a viewpoint near the falls. Go on a warm spring day, when the creek is in full flow and the chaparral is in bloom.

■ DESCRIPTION

From the 210 Freeway in Claremont, take Exit 52 for Base Line Road. Go west on Base Line 0.2 mile, then turn right (north) on Padua Avenue. In 1.8 miles, turn right onto Mount Baldy Road. Follow it 11.7 miles to Manker Flats, where you can park along the road (GPS N34° 15.966' W117° 37.614').

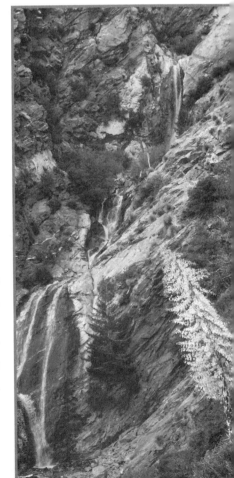

From Manker Flats, walk west through a gate and up a service road past some cabins. In 0.5 mile, the road makes a hairpin turn. This is the best viewpoint for San Antonio Falls. If you want a closer view, you can follow a narrow and tenuous dirt trail 150 yards to the base of the falls (GPS N34° 16.286' W117° 38.047'). Rock climbers sometimes practice alongside the falls.

The three tiers of San Antonio Falls

VARIATION Canyoneers could follow San Antonio Creek up the falls all the way to the Sierra Club ski hut, but this involves some fourth-class climbing, and most parties will want a rope. Stay left of the first waterfall and then right of the next ones. The walking then eases until you reach another waterfall just below the ski hut. Climb loose rock on the left side or bushwhack up the steep slope farther left. Unprepared parties have required rescue from this steep canyon.

■ Hike 92 MOUNT BALDY VIA DEVILS BACKBONE ↗ 🯅

HIKE LENGTH 6 miles out-and-back; 2,300' elevation gain
DIFFICULTY Moderate
SEASON June–October
MAP Tom Harrison *Angeles High Country*
PERMIT Ski-lift fee

■ FEATURES

Saint Anthony of Padua, a 13th-century Franciscan priest and miracle worker, is well represented in Southern California. His name crowns the San Gabriel Mountains—Mount San Antonio. Legend has it that the title was bestowed by the padres of Mission San Gabriel in the 1790s. Early American miners, digging in upper San Antonio Canyon in the 1870s, dubbed the peak an earthier Old Baldy for its barren, roundish summit. Although the U.S. Board on Geographic Names has decreed Mount San Antonio as official, Old Baldy and Mount Baldy are still favorites of most sightseers and hikers today.

Massive Mount San Antonio—or Old Baldy if you prefer—is the grand climax of the 50-mile backbone of the San Gabriels. No other peak in the range rises to challenge its 10,064-foot elevation. From its summit, you look over a good part of Southern California: an expanse of mountain, desert, and coastal lowland. On those rare days when haze does not muddy the atmosphere, the hiker on its boulder-strewn top can make out the tawny ramparts of the southern High Sierra, 160 miles in the distance.

Old Baldy is a huge mountain by Southern California standards. Its sprawling gray bulk overwhelms lesser summits and makes up for any lack of sharp relief. Long descending ridges and broad slopes of disintegrating

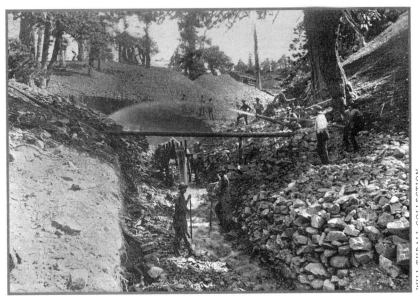

Hydraulic mining at Hocumac Mine near Baldy Notch, circa 1894

WILL THRALL COLLECTION

granitic rock drop far down into shadowy canyons. Among the folds of its granite robes are sylvan dells where sparkling streams and waterfalls rush downward and ferns grow lush in the shade of pines and cedars. Its higher slopes are dotted with lodgepole and limber pines. Some pines stand tall and erect, proud sentinels of the ridgetops; others are bent and gnarled by nature's high-altitude fury, forming grotesque shapes. All contribute to the elegance, order, and beauty of the alpine landscape.

We will probably never know who made the first ascent of Mount San Antonio. Serrano Indians, who knew the great mountain as Joat—their word for snow—crossed the San Antonio/Lytle Creek Divide (Baldy Notch) centuries before the arrival of the white man, and they may have walked the short distance to the top, although Native Americans of that day appear to have had little interest in "conquering" mountain peaks. Perhaps an early miner at the Banks (later Hocumac) Mine, just below Baldy Notch, scrambled to the summit. The earliest ascent on record was made by Louis Nell and a party of soldiers from the U.S. Army's Wheeler Survey on July 1, 1875.

The first name associated with the peak was that of William B. Dewey, who made the ascent in 1882. Dewey reported seeing no human trail up Baldy, but bears were plentiful and many bear trails contoured the higher

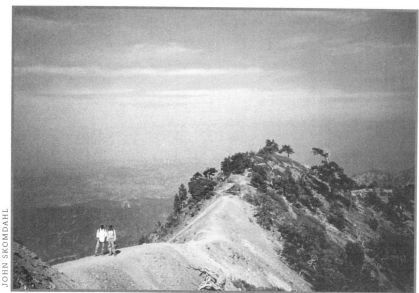

JOHN SKOMDAHL

Devil's Backbone Trail

slopes of the mountain. Dewey spent most of his life in San Antonio Canyon. From 1886 to 1888, he served as a mountain guide for Stoddard's Resort, leading many guests to the summit and back. In the summers of 1910–1912, he built and managed, with his wife, the Baldy Summit Inn. Located a mere 80 feet below the top, it was the most unique resort in the West. It consisted of two small stone buildings and several tents securely anchored against winds that sometimes reached gale force. Saddle horses and mules brought guests up from Camp Baldy (today's Mount Baldy Village) every day. Fire destroyed most of the camp in 1913, and Dewey never rebuilt it. He made a total of 133 ascents of Mount San Antonio. The last was in 1936, when he was 71 years old.

Old Baldy is a hiker's delight. The trail is well beaten and the grade easy (except the summit pitch). The thin air is invigorating, and vistas are breathtaking almost the entire distance. During summer and fall weekends, thousands of people, young and old alike, make the ascent. Probably no other Western mountain not reached by road is climbed by so many people.

This trip takes the easiest route to Mount Baldy's summit, using the ski lift to shave off the walk to Baldy Notch. The lift is typically open Friday–Sunday and holidays; call 909-982-0800 for current information, or buy discount tickets online at mtbaldyresort.com. Nevertheless, it can be a demanding hike at high altitude. If you'd prefer making the trip with no mechanical assistance, see Hike 94 for a great loop via Baldy Bowl and down the Devils Backbone.

Be alert for (and dress for) changing weather conditions. Summer thunderstorms are a possibility; beat a hasty retreat at the first sign of severe weather. And do not attempt an ascent of the mountain during snow season—which extends well into the warmer months most years—unless you are experienced in and equipped for winter mountaineering.

■ DESCRIPTION

From the 210 Freeway in Claremont, take Exit 52 for Base Line Road. Go west on Base Line for 0.2 mile, then turn right (north) on Padua Avenue. In 1.8 miles, turn right onto Mount Baldy Road. Follow it 11.7 miles up past Manker Flats to the Baldy ski-area parking, where your trip begins (GPS N34° 16.205' W117° 37.311').

Purchase your lift ticket and ride up to the restaurant at Baldy Notch. From Baldy Notch, follow the broad path east 150 yards to Desert View and a wooden sign pointing left (northwest) toward Mount Baldy. Turn left and proceed up the fire road, switchbacking up a broad slope shaded by Jeffrey and sugar pines, white firs, and incense cedars. The fire road ends at the top of a ski lift just before the razor-backed ridge known, for good reason, as the Devils Backbone. The trail proceeds along the backbone (people have slipped on ice here, so take care), climbs around the south slope of Mount Harwood through a thinning forest of lodgepole pines, emerges from the trees, and reaches a wind-battered saddle.

From here the trail steepens considerably as it ascends nearly bare slopes for the final 400 feet, passing a few stunted lodgepole pines here and there. Limber pines are curiously absent from the mountain, although they are found on the higher reaches of Mount Baden-Powell and adjoining summits. The top is a gently tapered expanse of boulders, barren of vegetation and commanding the broadest panorama in the San Gabriel Mountains (GPS N34° 17.351' W117° 38.780'). You could spend a starry windswept night up here. Return the way you came.

▪ Hike 93 MOUNT BALDY VIA BEAR RIDGE ↗ 🐐 🧍

HIKE LENGTH 10 miles one-way; 5,800' elevation gain
DIFFICULTY Strenuous
SEASON June–October
MAP Tom Harrison *Angeles High Country*
PERMIT N/A

▪ FEATURES

The great south ridge of Baldy rises in continuous welts from Cow Canyon Saddle to the summit, gaining more than 6,000 feet of elevation in 3 miles. The ridge begins in dense chaparral; passes through belts of Jeffrey and sugar pines, white firs, and lodgepole pines; and then terminates above timberline. Following the crest of this ridge most of the way, the Bear Canyon, or Old Mount Baldy, Trail (sometimes called the Bear Flat Trail) is one of the most strenuous hikes in the San Gabriels. Its 5,800 feet of elevation gain from Mount Baldy Village to the top rivals the Iron Mountain hike (see Hike 80) for the most of any footpath in the range. You could find dispersed camping at Bear Flat or on the summits of West Baldy or Baldy.

This is the hard way to do Old Baldy and is only for those in excellent physical condition. Veteran hikers call this a no-nonsense trail—direct, uphill all the way, and in some spots unbelievably steep. Those who complete this all-day trip are guaranteed to be exhausted at the finish.

Years ago, this was the main trail up Baldy. It was built in 1889 by Dr. B. H. Fairchild of Claremont and Fred Dell of Dell's Camp in San Antonio Canyon. The men envisioned a great astronomical observatory on the summit, but it was never built. In ensuing years, parties from Camp Baldy (today's Mount Baldy Village) would go up the trail on foot or horseback, watch the glorious sunset from the top, and stay the night at William B. Dewey's Baldy Summit Inn (see previous hike), returning the next day. With the extension of the road to the head of San Antonio Canyon and the construction of the Devils Backbone Trail by the Civilian Conservation Corps in 1935–1936, the old Bear Flat route fell into disuse. This is not a trail for beginners, although it remains easy to follow if you are physically—and temperamentally—inclined.

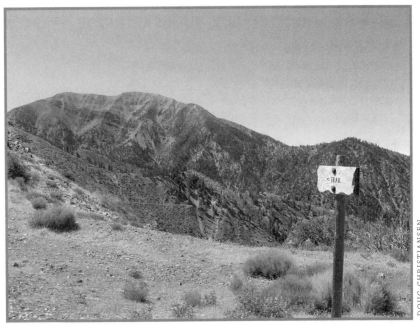

DOUG CHRISTIANSEN

Trail to Mount Baldy

■ DESCRIPTION

This trip requires a 4-mile car or bicycle shuttle. To leave your getaway vehicle at Manker Flats, take Exit 52 from the 210 Freeway onto Base Line Road. Go west on Base Line for 0.2 mile, then turn right (north) on Padua Avenue. In 1.8 miles, turn right onto Mount Baldy Road. Follow it 11.7 miles to Manker Flats, where there is roadside parking (GPS N34° 15.966' W117° 37.614'). Then drive or pedal 4 miles back down the road to the Mount Baldy Trout Ponds, where you'll find plenty of parking across the road above Mount Baldy Village (GPS N34° 14.322' W117° 39.238').

Walk down to Mount Baldy Village and turn right onto Bear Canyon Road just below the visitor center. Hiker parking is not permitted along this road. Walk up Bear Canyon Road past numerous cabins for 0.4 mile to its end, where you turn onto the signed Bear Canyon Trail. The trail switchbacks up slopes shaded by live oaks and firs to Bear Flat, a small mountain meadow clothed in a carpet of lush grass, at 2.1 miles. You might find water here, the last along the route. This area burned in the 2008 Bighorn Fire.

Above Bear Flat, the trail zigzags steeply through shadeless chaparral, the most unpleasant part of the trip on a hot day, to the crest of the south ridge. Here, amid cool stands of pines and firs, the view opens to the west, across the deep canyons of the San Gabriel watershed to the Mount Wilson–Strawberry Peak–Charlton Flat country. The trail now ascends the ridgeline, over an extremely steep and loose-footed pitch known in the old days as Hardscrabble, to The Narrows, a razor-backed saddle at 9,200 feet. After crossing the bare saddle, the route enters an open forest of weather-toughened lodgepole pines, traverses the east slope of West Baldy, emerges above timberline, and climbs finally to the 10,064-foot summit for a top-of-the-world vista at 6.4 miles (GPS N34° 17.351' W117° 38.780').

Descend to Manker Flat via the Devils Backbone or Ski Hut Trails (see next hike). A satisfying but most exhausting day's walk!

■ Hike 94 MOUNT BALDY LOOP ↻ 🐕 🏃

HIKE LENGTH 10-mile loop; 3,900' elevation gain
DIFFICULTY Strenuous
SEASON June–October
MAP Tom Harrison *Angeles High Country*
PERMIT N/A

■ FEATURES

This is the most direct way to Mount Baldy's summit, but it's also the steepest. It's trail all the way, but some sections of the footpath, particularly from Baldy Bowl to the top, are loose and not well maintained. Nevertheless, this is one of the most scenic and historical hikes in the San Gabriels. You pass near the remains of the old Gold Ridge Mine, worked in the 1890s; the Sierra Club's San Antonio Ski Hut; Baldy Bowl, where Southern California skiing was born in the 1930s; and, near the top, the site of Baldy Summit Inn, once the highest trail resort in the range. You make a loop by descending the scenic Devils Backbone and walking down the ski-area service road.

You should be in good physical condition, wear lug-soled boots, and tote plenty of water—the only sure source of it is a small stream you cross at the edge of Baldy Bowl, and even this may disappear by summer's end in years of below-average rainfall. This route is deceptively dangerous when icy,

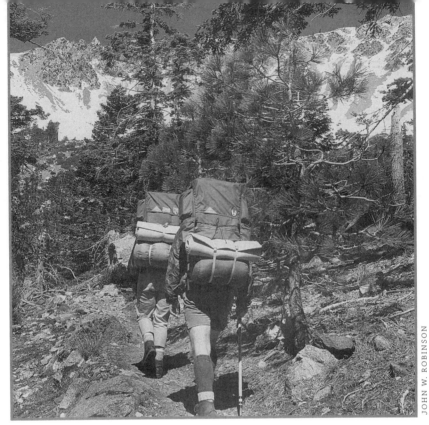

Backpackers at Baldy Bowl

and only experienced mountaineers with an ice ax, crampons, and proper skills should attempt it under winter or spring conditions.

■ DESCRIPTION

From the 210 Freeway in Claremont, take Exit 52 for Base Line Road. Go west on Base Line 0.2 mile, then turn right (north) on Padua Avenue. In 1.8 miles, turn right onto Mount Baldy Road. Follow it 11.7 miles to Manker Flats, where you can park alongside the road (GPS N34° 15.966' W117° 37.614').

Walk past the locked gate and up the ski-area service road, passing a fine view of San Antonio Falls at the first switchback, 0.5 mile. At 0.9 mile, look for the Baldy Bowl Trail, which begins steeply on your left. (There is no sign here, and it is easy to miss.) The trail climbs at a steady, steep grade up the east slope of upper San Antonio Canyon, through an open forest of Jeffrey and then lodgepole pines. On a sloping bench to your left, 1.25 miles up and about 100 yards off the trail, are the stone foundations of the Gold Ridge Mine, worked from 1897 to 1904. Reach the lower edge of Baldy Bowl at 2.4 miles. To your right, 50 feet away, is the Sierra Club's San Antonio Ski

Hut, built in 1935, burned in 1936, and rebuilt in 1937. Use of the hut is by reservation only, through the Angeles Chapter of the Sierra Club. Backpackers without reservations are invited to camp in the so-called Rock Garden, about 200 yards southwest of the hut.

You go left as your trail drops down to the trickling headwaters of San Antonio Creek, which has the only sure water en route. The water is icy cold and delicious, but it should be purified before drinking (as should all water in the San Gabriels). The trail contours through a boulder field across the lower edge of Baldy Bowl, a skier's delight in winter. Beyond, you reenter the lodgepole forest and zigzag steeply up to Mount Baldy's great southeast ridge. The north-facing slope holds ice after the rest of the trail has melted out. Your footpath ascends the ridgeline; passes just left of some small rock gendarmes; reaches the site of William Dewey's Baldy Summit Inn (open for hardy guests during the summers of 1910–1913); and finally arrives on the broad, barren summit of Mount San Antonio (10,064'), 4.0 steep miles from the start (GPS N34° 17.351' W117° 38.780').

After enjoying the summit, follow the Devils Backbone Trail down the east ridge of Baldy. Beware that five trails depart the summit ridge and that many hikers have taken the wrong one, especially when visibility is

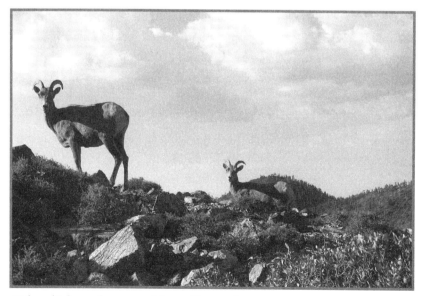

Nelson bighorn sheep near Mount Harwood

poor. The spectacular trail passes along the south side of Mount Harwood and then follows a knife-edge ridge down to the ski area at Baldy Notch (7,800') at 7.0 miles. All that remains is an easy 3.3-mile walk down the service road to Manker Flats. If your knees are complaining, you can buy a ticket down the ski lift instead.

■ Hike 95 STOCKTON FLAT TO BALDY NOTCH 🡕 🐐 ⊕

HIKE LENGTH 8 miles out-and-back; 1,700' elevation gain
DIFFICULTY Moderate
SEASON June–October
MAP Tom Harrison *Angeles High Country*
PERMIT N/A

■ FEATURES

Note: Check with the U.S. Forest Service (fs.usda.gov/angeles) about road conditions before attempting this hike. At the time of this writing, a high-clearance, four-wheel-drive vehicle was required. The road sometimes washes out completely.

Stockton Flat lies at the head of Lytle Creek, in a sloping bowl ringed by lofty peaks and ridges. This is the backyard of the San Antonio country, close under the gray mantle of Old Baldy itself. In the shadow of the massive mountain, snow lingers longer than in other parts of the range, providing coolness and moisture for handsome stands of pines and firs.

The flat was named for W. H. Stockton, who filed a timber claim here back in the 1880s. But apparently he did no cutting and never received a patent, and the flat reverted to the national forest. Despite the ravages of a series of wildfires, it remains quite appealing and serves as a jumping-off point for this backdoor approach to Mount Baldy.

This trip offers a different route to the Mount Baldy country, one that few of the multitude of Baldy hikers ever attempt. A steep dirt road, built originally in the 1890s to provide access to the Hocumac gold mine just over the ridge from Baldy Notch, climbs up the back side of the Baldy–Telegraph Ridge to the notch. This hiking trip takes you up this old mountain byway and offers you several options. It's a pleasant summer outing when the air is crisp but not biting, and the open forest offers both shade and sunshine. The

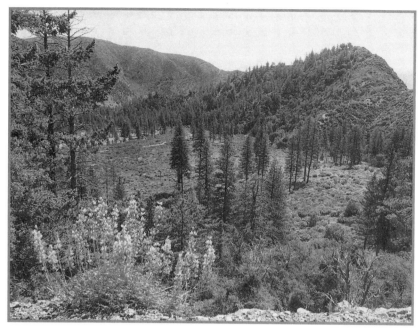

Stockton Flat

drive to the trailhead may be half the adventure. If you have time, consider spending a night at one of the secluded first-come, first-served yellow-post campsites along Forest Road 3N06.

■ DESCRIPTION

From I-15 in Nealeys Corner, take Exit 119 for Sierra Avenue. Follow Sierra Avenue north 11.3 miles as it becomes Lytle Creek Road and leads through Lytle Creek Village to the end of pavement. Continue on FR 3N06 for 3.9 miles, crossing the rocky wash bed and passing four excellent yellow-post campsites. A high-clearance vehicle such as a pickup truck is recommended, as there are several bad spots that could pose a problem for low-slung standard vehicles. The last mile might be faster to walk than drive. Park outside the locked gate on Stockton Flat (GPS N34° 17.719' W117° 36.058').

From the flat, walk up the poor dirt road, going left (south) at a junction, and wind steeply up the mountainside above Coldwater Canyon. As you gain elevation, vistas open up to the north and east, across the Lytle Creek and Cajon Pass country. Notice the parallel northwest–southeast orientation of the topography, following the line of California's greatest fault, the

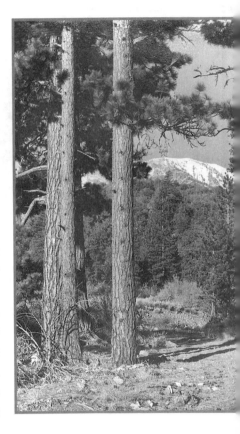

Old Baldy from Stockton Flat
C. W. MCLAUGHLIN

San Andreas. Finally, there is one long switchback, and you round the head of Coldwater Canyon's north fork to Baldy Notch, 3.8 miles from the start (GPS N34° 16.523' W117° 36.518'). You can visit Top of the Notch restaurant, and then return the way you came.

VARIATIONS You can take the Devils Backbone Trail to Baldy's summit (Hike 92); take the trail south over "the three Ts"—Thunder, Telegraph, and Timber—to Icehouse Saddle, where more options open up (see next hike); or, if you can arrange to be picked up in San Antonio Canyon, take the ski lift or hike down the fire road to Manker Flat, where you meet the paved road.

■ Hike 96 THE THREE TS 🡕 🐐 🥾

> **HIKE LENGTH** 10 miles one-way; 2,000' elevation gain, 4,800' elevation loss
> **DIFFICULTY** Moderate
> **SEASON** June–October
> **MAP** Tom Harrison *Angeles High Country*
> **PERMIT** Post Adventure Pass, or park outside fee area. Lift ticket required if using the ski lift.

■ FEATURES

Between Baldy Notch and Icehouse Saddle, at the head of the great horseshoe ridge that encircles upper San Antonio Canyon, are three summits rising more than 8,000 feet—Thunder Mountain (8,587'), Telegraph Peak (8,985'), and Timber Mountain (8,303'). Mountaineers know these forested knobs as the three Ts. This trip traverses over *or* around these three summits—depending on whether you are a peak bagger—on good trail.

This is ideal summer hiking country. The well-beaten ridge trail offers continuous vistas as it zigzags over crests and across saddles, and through open stands of pines, firs, and cedars. Snow patches linger in sheltered recesses well into the warmer months. The high-mountain air is cool, clear, and clean, with seldom a trace of the urban-generated murkiness that clogs lungs at lower elevations. From Telegraph Peak, the climax of the trip, the desert view rivals the one from Baldy. (Telegraph's name dates from the 1890s, when government surveyors installed a heliograph on the summit and signaled to cohorts on Mount Wilson, 22 air miles away.)

This trip covers a lot of high country, but you get a head start by taking the ski lift to Baldy Notch. From there it's 1,100 feet up Telegraph and then downhill most of the rest of the way to the Icehouse Canyon parking area. For this reason, it can be classified as moderate. If you want to do it the other way, add almost 2,000 feet more climbing and consider it strenuous. You can find dispersed camping along the ridge, but you must haul your own water.

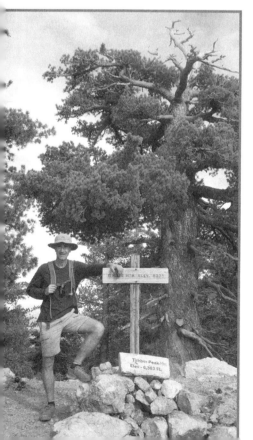

Timber Mountain

■ DESCRIPTION

This trip requires a short car shuttle. From the 210 Freeway in Claremont, take Exit 52 for Base Line Road. Go west on Base Line 0.2 mile, then turn right (north) on Padua Avenue. In 1.8 miles, turn right onto Mount Baldy Road. Follow it 9 miles up to Icehouse Canyon and leave a vehicle at the trailhead on the right (GPS N34° 15.007' W117° 38.163'). Continue 3 miles up hairpin turns past Manker Flats to the Baldy ski-area parking (GPS N34° 16.205' W117° 37.311').

Buy a one-way ticket and ride the ski lift to Baldy Notch (operated weekends and holidays all year). An alternate way to the notch, one that adds 3.5 miles and 1,500 feet of elevation gain to the hike, is to walk the fire road from Manker Flats, passing San Antonio Falls.

From Top of the Notch restaurant, walk east about 150 yards to Desert View, where you pick up the fire road leading southeast up Gold Ridge. Follow the fire road 1.4 miles to the base of a ski run leading to the top of Thunder Mountain. Don't climb directly up the slope; instead, look for a trail branching off to the right. Follow the trail as it traverses and climbs around the south ridge of Thunder Mountain (GPS N34° 15.915' W117° 36.361') and then drops 500 feet to a saddle. From here the trail switchbacks steeply 800 feet to the top of Telegraph Peak ridge at 2.6 miles. Turn left (northeast) and follow the ridgetop 0.2 mile to the summit (GPS N34° 15.702' W117° 35.908'). Return to the main trail and follow it south along the ridge—downhill except where you climb briefly around the west slope of Timber Mountain. At 5.1 miles, a use trail makes a short detour to the summit of Timber (GPS N34° 14.706' W117° 35.620'). Continue the descent to Icehouse Saddle at 6.2 miles. Then turn right (west) and descend the Icehouse Canyon Trail (see next hike) to the Icehouse Canyon parking area.

■ Hike 97 ICEHOUSE SADDLE FROM ICEHOUSE CANYON 🥾 🐕 🚶

HIKE LENGTH 7 miles out-and-back; 2,600' elevation gain
DIFFICULTY Moderate
SEASON June–October
MAP Tom Harrison *Angeles High Country*
PERMIT Post Adventure Pass, or park outside fee area.

■ FEATURES

Icehouse Canyon is the hikers' gateway to the eastern high country and the Cucamonga Wilderness. Its broad, V-shaped portal leads east from San Antonio Canyon 1.5 miles north of Mount Baldy Village and climbs 2,600 feet to Icehouse Saddle, a prominent gap on the great Telegraph–Ontario Ridge. The saddle is a major trail junction, with routes leading in five directions.

For hikers seeking a moderate outing, the trip upcanyon to Icehouse Saddle is rewarding. You pass through some of the finest stands of incense cedars in the range, and the ponderosa, Jeffrey, and sugar pines are healthy

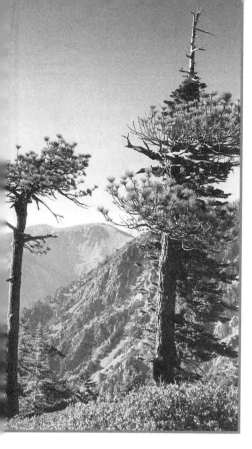

*Mount Baldy from Icehouse
Canyon Trail*
BETTY DESSERT

and towering. From the saddle you look into the inviting Cucamonga Wilderness country and down over the Lytle Creek drainage.

Legend has it that the magnificent cedar beams for Mission San Gabriel were cut in the canyon and then laboriously dragged down to the lowland by oxen teams. For years it was known as Cedar Canyon (now the name for a tributary of Icehouse Canyon). The present name dates from the 1860s, when an ice plant in the lower canyon supplied ice to valley residents.

The lower reaches of the canyon are dotted with private cabins. Once, there were many more; the big flood of 1938 wreaked havoc here, as it did in other canyons of the range. Today the boulder-strewn floor of Icehouse Canyon bears testimony to nature's torrential fury.

■ DESCRIPTION

From the 210 Freeway in Claremont, take Exit 52 for Base Line Road. Go west on Base Line for 0.2 mile, then turn right (north) on Padua Avenue. In 1.8 miles, turn right onto Mount Baldy Road. Follow it 9 miles to Ice House Canyon Road on the right, where you'll reach a large trailhead parking area that can fill early on the weekends (GPS N34° 15.007' W117° 38.163'). You may find overflow parking on the shoulder of Mount Baldy Road.

Walk up the trail that starts just to the right of the parking area. The trail climbs gently through a forest of oaks, big-cone Douglas-firs, and incense cedars as you pass many cabins. You reach a junction in 1.0 mile. To your left, the Chapman Trail climbs in gentle switchbacks 0.3 mile to an excellent trail camp at Cedar Glen and continues on an airy high route along the precipitous north slope of the canyon to a junction with the main Icehouse Canyon Trail, 5 miles from the start. This trip, however, follows the main trail, which continues straight ahead, passes a cluster of cabins, follows the creek another 0.5 mile, and then crosses it. The creek disappears as you climb steadily, under an open forest of pines and incense cedars, and enter Cucamonga Wilderness, marked with a large wooden sign. At 2.2 miles you reach Columbine Spring, a small seepage of icy-cold water just below the trail. This is the last water en route. Beyond, the trail switchbacks up under a shady canopy of tall pines and firs, passes a junction with the upper end of the Chapman Trail, and reaches Icehouse Saddle, 3.3 miles from the start (GPS N34° 14.352' W117° 35.665').

Take a good look, and then return the way you came.

VARIATIONS From the saddle, you can either turn left (north) and follow the trail that climbs around the west slope of Timber Mountain and over Telegraph Peak before dropping to Baldy Notch (see previous hike); turn hard right (southwest) and take the lateral trail to Kelly's Camp and Ontario Peak (see next hike); go right (southeast) on the trail that contours around the east slopes of Bighorn Peak to Cucamonga Saddle, and then climb the north face of Cucamonga Peak (see Hike 99); or drop eastward down the Middle Fork Trail to Lytle Creek (see Hike 100). Returning from the saddle via the Chapman Trail adds 1.5 miles, making a good semiloop trip. Whichever option you take, you are sure to travel through some of the finest high country in the range.

■ Hike 98 ONTARIO PEAK 🡕 🐕 🚶

HIKE LENGTH 12 miles out-and-back; 3,800' elevation gain
DIFFICULTY Strenuous
SEASON June–October
MAP Tom Harrison *Angeles High Country*
PERMIT Post Adventure Pass or park outside fee area. Free first-come, first-served camping.

■ FEATURES

From Icehouse Saddle, the long, multi-humped Ontario Ridge juts southwestward, standing above 8,000 feet for some 2 miles, separating the San Antonio from the Cucamonga watershed. Blanketing the upper north slopes of the ridge is a lush forest—rather dense in sheltered recesses, thinning

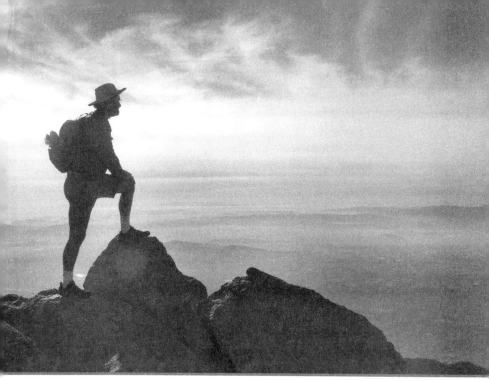

Surveying the Inland Empire from Ontario Peak   WERNER ZORMAN

out on the crests—of white firs; Jeffrey and sugar pines; and, higher up, lodgepole pines.

The Ontario Peak Trail traverses this ridge, staying just on the north side of the crest, from Icehouse Saddle to the 8,693-foot summit. En route, it visits Kelly's Camp—established as a mining prospect by John Kelly in 1905, turned into a trail resort by Henry Delker in 1922, and now an unimproved wilderness campsite.

You can do this trip in one day as a rather strenuous up-and-back hike, or you can make it a more leisurely outing by staying the night at Kelly's Camp. Just beyond the camp is a small spring, flowing in early season but sometimes drying up in late summer and fall. If it's been a dry year, you should pack all your own water. Open fires are prohibited at wilderness camps.

■ DESCRIPTION

From the 210 Freeway in Claremont, take Exit 52 for Base Line Road. Go west on Base Line for 0.2 mile, then turn right (north) on Padua Avenue. In 1.8 miles, turn right onto Mount Baldy Road. Follow it 9 miles to Ice House

Canyon Road on the right, where you'll reach a large trailhead parking area that can fill early on the weekends (GPS N34° 15.007' W117° 38.163'). You may find overflow parking on the shoulder of Mount Baldy Road.

Walk up the trail 3.3 miles to Icehouse Saddle (see previous hike). From the saddle, take the far-right fork, traveling southwest across the forested slopes. A mile of level and uphill walking through the forest brings you to Kelly's Camp at 4.2 miles (GPS N34° 14.033' W117° 36.274'). Your trail climbs around the left side of the wilderness campsite; it then circles right, climbs to the top of the ridge, intersects the short lateral trail leading left to Bighorn Peak, and turns west. You walk through a lodgepole forest (much of it burned in the 2003 Grand Prix Fire), passing just to the right of two false summits, and finally surmount Ontario Peak at 5.8 miles (GPS N34° 13.662' W117° 37.441').

Enjoy the superb view from the top, and then return the same way.

■ Hike 99 CUCAMONGA PEAK 🡕 🐕 🚶

HIKE LENGTH 12 miles out-and-back; 4,000' elevation gain
DIFFICULTY Strenuous
SEASON June–October
MAP Tom Harrison *Angeles High Country*
PERMIT Post Adventure Pass, or park outside fee area. Free Cucamonga Wilderness Permit required; apply online at tinyurl.com/cucamongawp. Group size limited to 12.

■ FEATURES

The Cucamonga Wilderness, enlarged to its present 12,781 acres when Congress passed the California Wilderness Act in 1984, is a high subalpine region of 8,000-foot peaks and deep canyons—pine-forested, precipitous, and relatively isolated. This superb, nearly pristine high country extends from upper Icehouse Canyon and Thunder Mountain Ridge eastward some 4 miles to Grizzly Ridge, the upper Middle Fork of Lytle Creek, and rugged Cucamonga Peak. It is the only wilderness in Southern California that encompasses parts of two national forests—Angeles and San Bernardino.

The 8,859-foot Cucamonga Peak is the eastern citadel of the range. Its steep battlements rise abruptly from Cucamonga Saddle on one side and San Sevaine Ridge on the other, offering nothing but discouragement to fainthearted and out-of-condition hikers.

The only easy access to Cucamonga Peak and its surrounding wilderness is via Icehouse Canyon and Saddle. A well-marked trail contours around the east slope of Bighorn Peak and zigzags steeply up the north side of Cucamonga. It's a long hike, but the view from the summit—taking in the eastern end of the range, the San Bernardino Valley, and the mountains beyond—is well worth the effort. Dispersed camping is possible near the summit

■ DESCRIPTION

From the 210 Freeway in Claremont, take Exit 52 for Base Line Road. Go west on Base Line for 0.2 mile, then turn right (north) on Padua Avenue. In 1.8 miles, turn right onto Mount Baldy Road. Follow it 9 miles to Ice House Canyon Road on the right, where you'll reach a large trailhead parking area that can fill early on the weekends (GPS N34° 15.007' W117° 38.163'). You may find overflow parking on the shoulder of Mount Baldy Road.

Walk up the trail 3.3 miles to Icehouse Saddle (see Hike 97). From the saddle, turn right (southeast), noting trails to Ontario Peak (right) and Middle Fork Lytle Creek (left), and follow the Cucamonga Peak Trail as it contours through open stands of pines and white firs around the east slopes of

The Diving Board on Cucamonga Peak

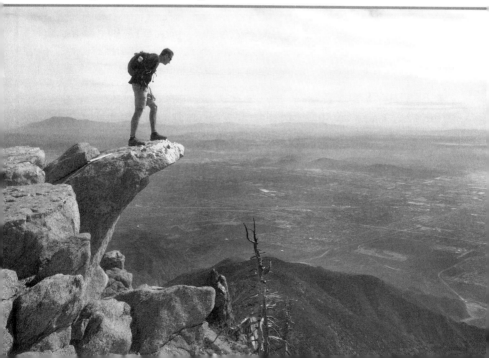

Bighorn Peak and gains Cucamonga Saddle at 4.3 miles. Here, you can look down into the wild, trailless gorge of Cucamonga Canyon. (See ropewiki.com for a memorable technical descent.) The trail then switchbacks steeply up the north face of Cucamonga Peak to within 200 feet of the summit and then turns east. Follow the well-worn spur to the summit at 5.7 miles (GPS N34° 13.346' W117° 35.109'). Return the same way.

VARIATION If you have more oomph, you can continue east on the trail from Cucamonga to Etiwanda Peak (GPS N34° 13.703' W117° 34.351'). This adds 2.2 miles round-trip with 700 feet of elevation gain. The Etiwanda Peak Trail continues 5 more miles down to abandoned Big Tree Campground, but this area burned in the 2003 Grand Prix Fire, and the trail is unmaintained and deteriorating.

■ Hike 100 ICEHOUSE SADDLE FROM LYTLE CREEK 🥾 🐕 🚶

HIKE LENGTH 12 miles out-and-back; 3,600' elevation gain

DIFFICULTY Strenuous (1 day); moderate (2 days)

SEASON June–October

MAP Tom Harrison *Angeles High Country*

PERMIT Post Adventure Pass. Free Cucamonga Wilderness Permit at Lytle Creek Ranger Station or online at tinyurl.com/cucamongawp. Group size limited to 12. Permit required to camp at Commanche, Third Stream Crossing, or Stone House Crossing. Free first-come, first-served camping.

■ FEATURES

The 12,781-acre Cucamonga Wilderness covers the eastern end of the San Antonio high country, where the mountains are abruptly cut off by the earth-grinding cleaver of the San Andreas Fault. The terrain is as steep and rugged as any in the range. Razor-backed ridges and broken battlements of grayish, decomposing granite plunge downward from Telegraph and Cucamonga Peaks to meet the strange slanting valleys of the great fault.

This trip takes the eastern approach to the wilderness, climbing up the Middle Fork of Lytle Creek through the heart of the wild area to Icehouse Saddle on its western boundary. Along the way are three wilderness campsites (formerly trail camps) for overnight stay—Stone House, Third Crossing, and Comanche. You start in semiarid chaparral, progress upward

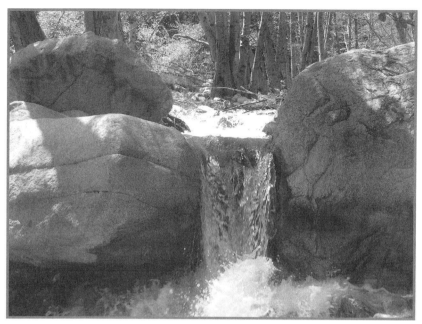

Lytle Creek

through belts of big-cone Douglas-firs and Jeffrey pines, and end up in the cool high country of lodgepole pines and white firs. From Icehouse Saddle, one of the major trail junctions in the range, you are presented with numerous options.

This is not a hike for beginners. Although passable, the trail is steep and primitive in places, with several eroded and exposed sections requiring extra care. Wear lug-soled boots, and don't do it alone; this is some of the loneliest mountain country in the range.

You stand a good chance of having the canyon all to yourself—99% of hikers who enter the wilderness do so from the gentler western side, via Icehouse Canyon or Baldy Notch. If you're lucky, you may spot a timid member of the Cucamonga herd of Nelson bighorn sheep—once plentiful but now rare in these mountains. This is one of the few islands of subalpine wilderness left in Southern California. Explore it, enjoy it, and protect it.

■ **DESCRIPTION**

From I-15, take Exit 119 north for Sierra Avenue, which becomes Lytle Creek Road. Proceed 4.6 miles to the Lytle Creek Ranger Station, where you can pick up your free Cucamonga Wilderness Permit. Continue 1.7 miles, then turn left onto Middle Fork Road, which soon becomes fair dirt Forest Road 2N58 (a high-clearance vehicle may be required). In 2.9 miles, reach the trailhead parking at the end of the road (GPS N34° 15.222' W117° 32.423').

Walk up the trail as it climbs the north slope above the streambed. In 0.5 mile you round a point and reach a trail junction. Go right, staying high on the slope; the left branch descends to the creek and Stone House wilderness campsite (GPS N34° 15.098' W117° 33.080'). You pass through stands of live oaks and big-cone Douglas-firs and reach an open, rocky area where the trail disappears, 2.3 miles from the start. Turn sharply left and cross the creek to Third Crossing wilderness campsite (GPS N34° 15.239' W117° 34.280'). (This was the third crossing of the Middle Fork via the historic trail routing; now it is the first crossing.) Above Third Crossing Camp, the trail ascends a sloping bench on the left (south) side of the creek, and then zigzags up the slope before leveling off just above the Middle Fork's south branch. There are several sections in this part of the trail that have been nearly washed out, making it the most difficult part of the hike. A pair of hiking poles would be most helpful here. You reach Comanche wilderness campsite, shaded by oaks, cedars, and firs, 4.0 miles up from the roadhead (GPS N34° 14.549' W117° 34.805'). You'll probably have Comanche all to yourself; it is one of the most isolated wilderness campsites in the San Gabriels. Don't expect to encounter any Comanches here; those Native Americans were natives of the southern Great Plains. From Comanche campsite, the trail climbs steeply west to the five-way trail junction of Icehouse Saddle at 5.7 miles (GPS N34° 14.352' W117° 35.665').

You have numerous options from Icehouse Saddle. You can return the way you came; you can take the trail west to Kelly's Camp and Ontario Peak (see Hike 98); you can go south on the Cucamonga Peak Trail (see previous hike); you can go north over the three Ts—Thunder Mountain, Telegraph Peak, and Timber Mountain (see Hike 96); or you can descend Icehouse Canyon to Mount Baldy Road (see Hike 97; this will require a long car shuttle).

OPPOSITE: *Marshall Canyon (see Hike 86)*

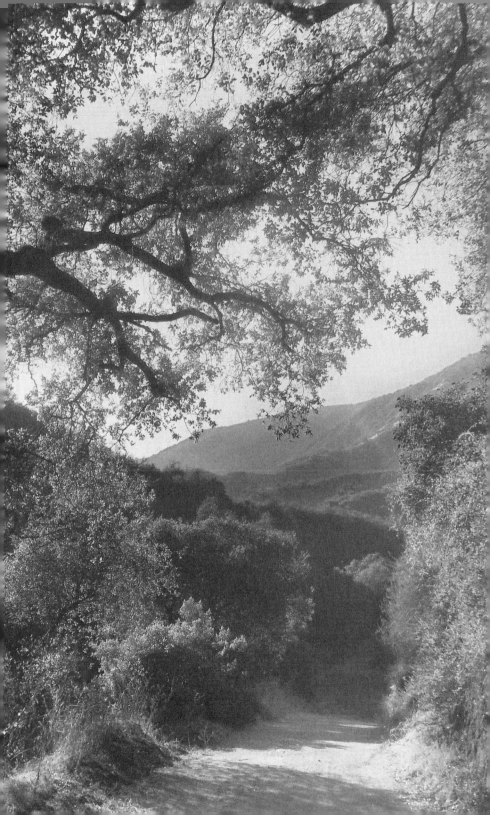

Appendix: Trails That Used to Be

DURING THE GREAT HIKING ERA (approximately 1895–1938), outdoor enthusiasts trekked by the thousands through the San Gabriels. With the building of the Angeles Crest Highway and other paved roads into the mountains, hiking interest declined, and many of these old pathways fell into disuse and disappeared. Others, not preempted by highway, are still in use today. Below are some of the historic trails of yesteryear that have faded or become virtually impassable.

ANGELES CREST TRAIL This famous footpath, now preempted by the Angeles Crest Highway, crossed the backbone of the mountains from Chilao to Islip Saddle, then descended the North Fork San Gabriel River to Coldwater Camp. A branch went from Islip Saddle down the South Fork of Big Rock Creek to the old Shoemaker Ranger Station. Hunters, anglers, and adventurers traveled it in great numbers from the 1890s into the 1930s. Today parts are gone completely, and other parts parallel the Angeles Crest Highway a few hundred feet above.

AZUSA–CAMP RINCON TRAIL When the San Gabriel River would flood in the old days, travel up the main canyon was virtually impossible. When this happened, visitors to Camp Rincon—a popular resort located where the present Rincon Ranger Station stands—took the high road over the mountains west of the river. Today the lower part of the old pathway is still passable; the upper section has been preempted by the Red Box–Rincon fire road.

BARLEY FLATS The trail to Barley Flats from Alder Creek on Big Tujunga Canyon Road burned in the 2009 Station Fire and was never rebuilt. It was reported impassable as of 2018.

BIGHORN RIDGE–OLD BALDY TRAIL In the early decades of the 20th century, Weber's Camp in Coldwater Canyon, a tributary of the East Fork San Gabriel River, was a popular trail resort. A trail was built from the camp up massive Bighorn Ridge to the summit of Baldy. With the demise of Weber's Camp in the 1920s, the trail was abandoned. It has now virtually disappeared.

CLIFF TRAIL This footpath between Mount Wilson and Mount Lowe Tavern was built in 1919, and for many years the stretch that crossed the south face of San Gabriel Peak was considered the most harrowing in the range. A misstep would send a hiker plunging 200 feet straight down. In 1942 the Mount Lowe Fire Road was blasted across the face, with a tunnel bypassing the sheer part. Hikers walking the fire road today, between Eaton and Markham Saddles, can see the remains of the old Cliff Trail traversing the rock face outside the tunnel.

DAGGER FLAT A mining road led from the Dillon Divide on Little Tujunga Road to the former Dutch Louie Flat Campground and on to Dutch Louie's tunnel and Dagger Flat. This area burned in the 2016 Sand Fire and is unmaintained and brushy.

DEER PARK–MONROVIA TRAIL Ben Overturff built this trail from Deer Park Lodge up the long southeast ridge of Monrovia Peak to the summit in 1914–1915. It fell into disrepair when Deer Park was abandoned after the 1938 flood.

EATON CANYON TRAIL No other canyon in the front range of the San Gabriels can compare with Eaton in ruggedness and inaccessibility. Access into the canyon now is from above, via the Idlehour Trail. Years ago, there was a cliff-hanging footpath up the canyon from Eaton Falls near the canyon entrance to Camp Idlehour. Many hikers were injured in falls from this precipitous trail. Today it is completely gone, and only experienced canyoneers with ropes, wet suits, and swift-water skills should venture here. See ropewiki.com for a route description.

ETIWANDA PEAK TRAIL The Etiwanda Peak Trail starts at the abandoned Joe Elliot Campground. The area burned in the 2003 Grand Prix Fire, and the trail has not received much maintenance. As of this writing, it is still passable but not in good enough shape to recommend for this book. Access is via a long drive up Forest Road 1N34 from Lytle Creek. The road is closed March 1–Labor Day, and a high-clearance vehicle is required. Brush impinging on the road may scratch your paint.

FALLS CREEK The Falls Creek Trail led from the Angeles Forest Highway just north of Hidden Springs Picnic Area to Big Tujunga Canyon Road. This area burned in the 2009 Station Fire, and the trail has not been rebuilt.

LONE TREE TRAIL Inventor Thaddeus S. C. Lowe built this steep trail from Rubio Pavilion up the divide between Rubio and Eaton Canyons to Panorama Point in the 1890s. Only one pine tree was passed en route, hence the trail's name. Today it is unmaintained but passable. You can gain the lower ridge from a spur off the Altadena Crest Trail or from either of two trails coming up from Rubio Canyon.

LOOKOUT MOUNTAIN TRAIL In 1913 the first fire lookout tower in Angeles National Forest was built, atop Lookout Mountain, which is a bump on Mount Baldy's great south ridge. A trail was constructed from Camp Baldy to Bear Flat, and then up to the summit. It became a favorite of Camp Baldy visitors because of the superb panorama available from Lookout Mountain. In 1927 the lookout was moved to nearby Sunset Peak, and the trail was abandoned. The area burned in the 2008 Bighorn Fire. The path leaving Bear Flat is obscure, but once you are established, it is generally possible to follow. Another route to Lookout Mountain from Cow Canyon Saddle is now blocked by a property owner. It is still possible to reach Lookout Mountain via a faint path from Bear Canyon to the saddle northwest of Peak 5,896.

LOOMIS RANCH TRAIL Like Colby Ranch, Loomis Ranch was beloved by hikers during the Great Hiking Era. This alder-shaded home of Captain Lester Loomis and his wife, Grace, located on Alder Creek west of Chilao, was the most remote of the trail resorts, but the popularity of Mrs. Loomis's chicken dinners and apple dumplings kept it well attended by visitors. Today Loomis Ranch is inaccessible to the public.

MONROVIA PEAK TRAIL This was once a favorite of Big Santa Anita Canyon hikers, going from Fern Lodge up the East Fork to Clamshell Ridge and on to the summit. Today the middle stretch from the East Fork up to the Clamshell fire road is completely overgrown and impassable.

PRAIRIE FORK A trail used to lead from Cabin Flat Campground down Prairie Fork to the East Fork San Gabriel River. The canyon burned in the 1997 Beiderbach Fire and is overgrown with thickets of thorny bushes, stinging nettles, and poison oak.

SAN DIMAS CANYON TRAIL San Dimas Canyon is now part of the San Dimas Experimental Forest, where various types of conifers are tested to determine their suitability to the Southern California mountains. Trails in and around the canyon are closed to the public.

SAWMILL MOUNTAIN RIDGE A trail led from the abandoned Atmore Meadows Campground on Sawmill Mountain Ridge into Bear Canyon and Gillette Mine. This area has received little use or maintenance in many years and has become faint and overgrown.

STURTEVANT TRAIL This once heavily trod footpath climbed from Sierra Madre over the ridge into Big Santa Anita and along the west slope to Sturtevant Camp. The lower third was made obsolete by the construction of the Chantry Flat Road in 1935 and is now eroded and blocked at both ends. The middle and upper stretches from Chantry Flat to Hoegees Trail Camp and on to Sturtevant are still passable and are described in Hike 37.

TOM LUCAS TRAIL Before the Station Fire, it was possible to make an excellent loop on Condor Peak by climbing the Condor Peak Trail from near Vogel Flat and descending the Tom Lucas Trail past Tom Lucas Trail Camp to the Trail Canyon Trail. This area burned in the 2009 Station Fire. The Condor Peak Trail has been repaired, but the upper portion of the Tom Lucas Trail is severely overgrown. As of 2018, it was still passable but involved long stretches of crawling through buckthorn and other brush. Trail crews hope to restore the trail one day.

TOM SLOAN TRAIL From its construction in 1923 until the demise of Mount Lowe Tavern in 1936, this route joining the tavern with Switzer's in the Arroyo Seco was a busy thoroughfare. In recent years, the stretch between the tavern and Tom Sloan Saddle became completely overgrown. However, volunteers from the Restoration Legacy Crew completely reworked this trail, as well as the portion into Millard Canyon, and it is in excellent shape again as of 2018.

Index

About the Author

DAVID HARRIS is a professor of engineering at Harvey Mudd College in Claremont, California. He is the author or coauthor of eight hiking guidebooks and five engineering textbooks. David grew up rambling around the Desolation Wilderness as a toddler in his father's pack and later roamed the High Sierra as a Boy Scout. As a Sierra Club trip leader, he organized mountaineering trips throughout the Sierra Nevada. Since 1999, David has been exploring the mountains and deserts of Southern California.

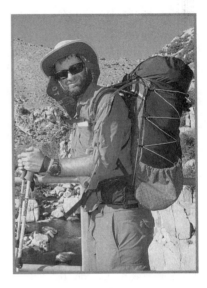

His other books for Wilderness Press are *101 Hikes in Southern California* (with Jerry Schad), *Afoot & Afield Los Angeles County* (with Jerry Schad), *Afoot & Afield Orange County* (with Jerry Schad), *Afoot & Afield Inland Empire, Day & Section Hikes Pacific Crest Trail: Southern California*, and *San Bernardino Mountain Trails* (with John W. Robinson). He is also a contributor to Wilderness Press's *Backpacking California*.

ABOUT THE ORIGINAL AUTHOR

JOHN W. ROBINSON (1929–2018) explored, backpacked, and climbed throughout the Mountain West for more than 50 years. His first guide, *Camping and Climbing in Baja* (now out of print), set the standard for guides to the Baja California mountains. In addition to the first seven editions of *Trails of the Angeles*, he authored or coauthored a number of the original Wilderness Press quadrangle guides, covering California's three major southern ranges: the San Gabriels, the San Bernardinos, and the San Jacintos. He also contributed numerous articles to *Westways, Desert Magazine, Southern California Quarterly, Overland Journal*, and *Summit*. If the mines of Southern California's mountains revealed gold and other precious minerals, they cannot compare to the treasure trove of information contained in this one man. His love for these forests, peaks, and wilderness areas is apparent on every page of his many works.